YOGA
OVER
50

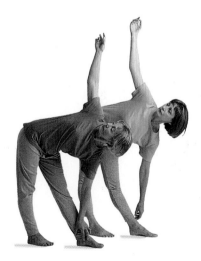

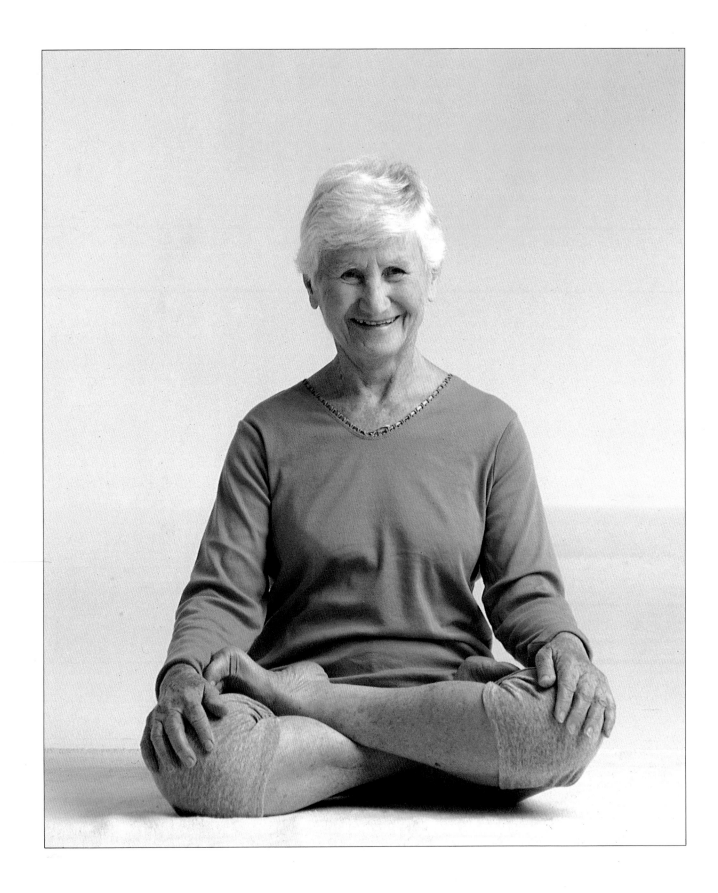

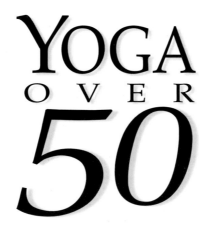

YOGA OVER 50

*The Way to Vitality, Health
and Energy in the Prime of Life*

by

MARY STEWART

Photography by
Sandra Lousada

A FIRESIDE Book
Published by SIMON & SCHUSTER INC.
New York London Toronto Sydney Tokyo Singapore

A FIRESIDE Book
Published by Simon & Schuster Inc.
Rockefeller Center
1230 Avenue of the Americas
New York, New York 10020

Color separations by Sele and Color , Bergamo, Italy.
Printed and bound in Hong Kong by Mandarin Offset.

10 9 8 7 6 5 4 3 2 1

Library of Congress Cataloging in Publication Data

Stewart, Mary (Mary E.)
Yoga over 50: the way to vitality, health and energy in later life/
by Mary Stewart:
photography by Sandra Lousada
p. cm.
"A Fireside book."
Includes index.
ISBN: 0-671-88510-3
1. Yoga, Hatha. 2. Exercise for the aged. I. Lousada, Sandra. II.
Title. III. Title: Yoga over 50.
RA781.7.S74 1994
613.7'046-dc20   93-41514
                        CIP

Created and designed by
Webster's Wine Price Guide Ltd,
Axe and Bottle Court, 70 Newcomen Street, London SE1 1YT

The exercises in this book are gentle and safe provided the
instructions are followed carefully. However, the publishers and
authors disclaim all liability in connection with the use of the
information in individual cases. If you have any doubts as to the
suitability of the exercises, consult a doctor.

C O N T E N T S

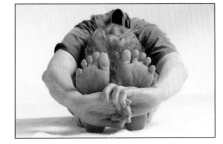

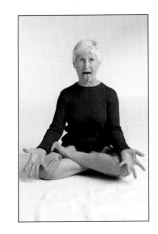

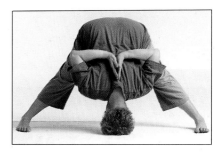

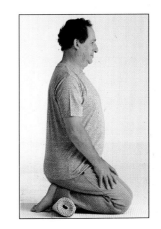

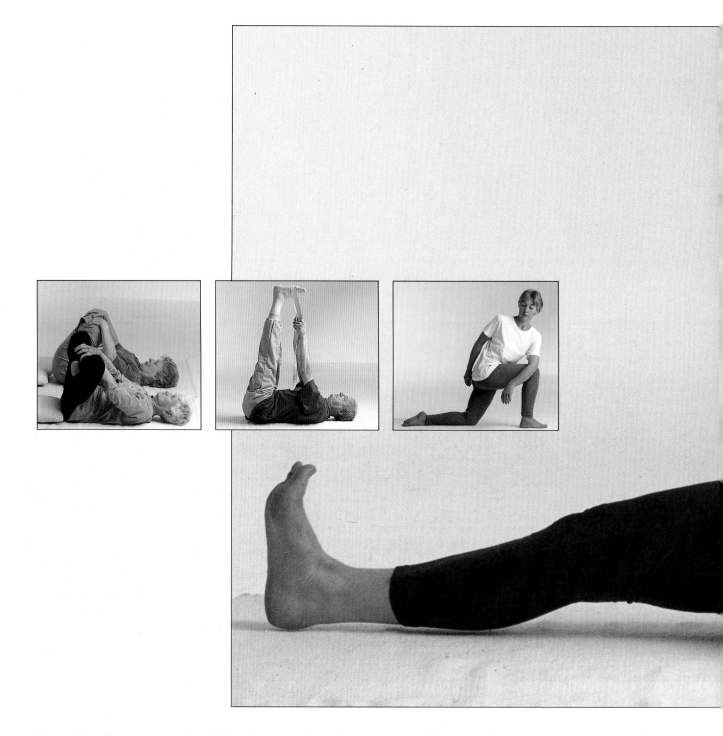

Yoga has been practiced for thousands of years. It is a system of bodily and mental exercises whose aim is freedom. Physically it promotes stability, energy, flexibility and relaxation. Mentally it promotes concentration, balance and tranquillity. In this book exercises are specially tailored to the needs and the particular problems of older people. Even short periods of regular, daily yoga practice can lead to positive changes in your quality of life, however old you are.

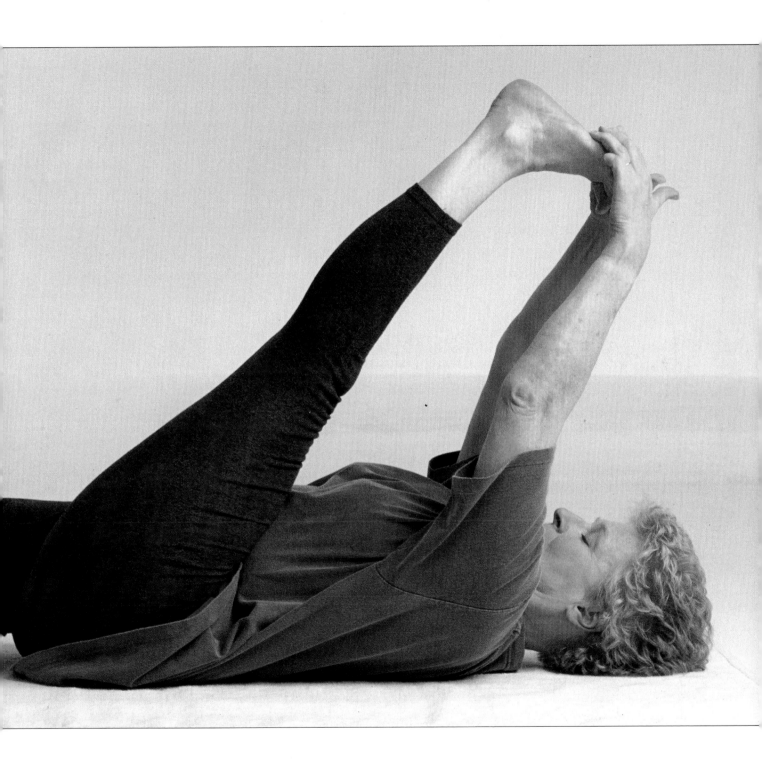

INTRODUCTION

PART ONE

WHAT YOGA IS ABOUT

GROWING OLDER IS AN INESCAPABLE fact of life. When we are young the physical capital we are born with seems inexhaustible. It is only when we reach middle age that we become more aware of the depletion of our natural stores of vitality. The good health and physical strength that we took for granted begin to show the results of wear and tear. The ageing process cannot be halted, but we do have the choice whether to conserve our health and make the most of our potential, or fritter away our energies. Yoga is about the first of these choices.

Making the most of age

In the latter half of the 20th century the energy and enthusiasm of youth are much sought after and the wisdom and experience of age tend to be undervalued. Not surprisingly the physical signs of ageing are something most people would prefer to hide, and someone who is "looking their age" is not thought to be doing too well. Together with the frantic search for eternal youth is the conviction that the inevitable accompaniment of age is the slow atrophy of retirement and the rest home. Such attitudes do not make it easy for us to approach the ageing process with any degree of sanity.

Yoga tradition is quite different: life is divided into four stages, each with a particular value and an essential role to play in a person's life. The first is the "student" or learning stage; the second is the "householder" or nest-building stage concerned with family and business responsibilities; the third is the "forest-dweller", or self-fulfillment stage, when domestic responsibilities tail off, and the fourth stage is the "wandering scholar" when the search for spiritual enlightenment becomes the main goal.

The aim at each stage is to realize the potential of that phase of life and the practice of yoga is part of the process.

In conventional forms of sport and exercise youth is considered a definite advantage. You peak at an early age and thereafter work hard to maintain your youthful strength and flexibility. This is not the case with yoga. The postures (*asanas*) and breathing (*pranayama*) are part of a system that aims to integrate mind, body and spirit. You learn the postures not by striving for perfection but by learning to "let go" the stiffness and tensions that inhibit movement, by learning how to move in rhythm with your breathing, and by realizing how the structure of your body is affected by gravity.

Yoga for fitness

Yoga is the oldest physical discipline there is. The original aim of the postures and breathing exercises was to bring stability and relaxation so that devotees could sit still and alert for long periods of meditation. Sitting still for long

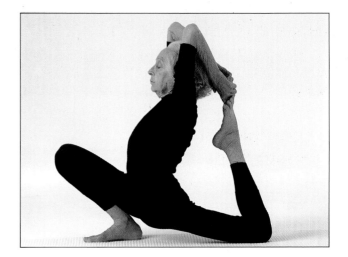

Yoga can be practiced at any age. This picture shows just how flexible someone in their 80s can be after many years' practice.

periods without getting stiff or tired is more demanding than you might think. It requires a considerable degree of physical fitness, attained only by keeping your body moving.

We need to move to stay healthy. Many of the complaints associated with ageing can be made less severe by keeping active and taking time to understand our body's need for movement as well as rest. Our minds also need concentration and silence. We might have to pace ourselves differently as we grow older, but we do not have to slide into inertia.

How you can benefit from yoga

Yoga postures (*asanas* in Sanskrit) stretch, extend and flex the spine. They exercise muscles and joints, keeping the body strong and supple. As they are done in conjunction with breathing, they stimulate circulation, digestion, nervous and endocrine systems, keeping you healthy and energetic. Yoga is quite different from popular modern ways of exercise. It does not aim to raise the heart-rate or work on specific muscle groups, or to help you to conform to a fashionable ideal. The postures release stiffness and tension, help to reestablish the inner balance of the spine, renew energy and restore health. Relaxation and breathing (pages 108–115) produce stability, reduce stress and put you in touch with your inner strength. This aspect of yoga becomes particularly important as you get older even if you are not practicing with any religious motive.

Yoga is for everyone

Yoga has stood the test of time. Practiced for thousands of years in the East, there are many tales of yogis living to a great age with all their physical and mental faculties intact. Today, since

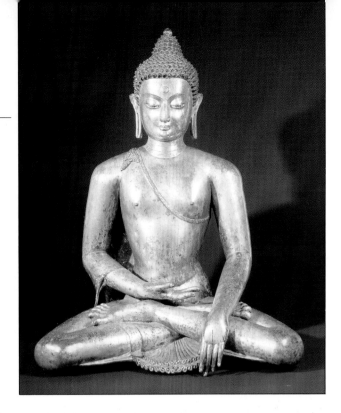

Statues of Buddha are often depicted sitting in the Lotus position; the skin is usually slightly taut from the divine energy within.

yoga has become popular in the West, there are plenty of witnesses to its benefits. The pictures in this book include people who have done yoga for some years and others who have only been practicing for a few months. Everyone who was photographed is over the age of 50 and some are in their 80s. All the postures shown have been practiced by people in their 80s, but this does not necessarily mean that all 80-year-olds will be able to do them.

Age is one of the least important factors in deciding which postures and breathing exercises you can and should practice. Inherited traits, habits of posture, previous experiences of exercise and many other factors affect the way our body is and how it functions. However, the physical, mental and spiritual boundaries are nowhere as near as we think they are.

Human beings have the most remarkable facility for change and regeneration throughout their lives. It is never too late to change bad habits and retune your body to use your energy more constructively.

HISTORY of YOGA

THE PRACTICE OF YOGA dates back thousands of years, to the dawn of civilization in the Indian subcontinent. Indian society has always absorbed ideas and beliefs from many diverse sources and the history of yoga is bound up in particular with the development of Hinduism and Buddhism. There is very little in the way of documentary evidence so the earliest history of yoga relies heavily on interpreting scraps of archeological data. Knowledge of yoga has, in any case, been passed on from teacher to pupil, resulting in a bewildering variety of strands influenced by different customs, myths and cultural developments.

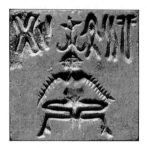

This ancient Indus Valley seal shows a yoga pose.

Early traces of yoga

The earliest evidence of yoga practice can be traced to the highly organized civilization that flourished in the Indus Valley thousands of years before the birth of Christ. Carved seals found in the ancient city of Mojendro-Daro and Harappa (in what is now Pakistan) depict figures seated in yoga positions (*see above*) and there is sculpture from this period suggesting the practice of meditation and the concept of inner energy (*prana*).

The decline of this civilization was followed by the Aryans migrating southward into India around 1500BC. The Aryans, who came from Central Asia, brought with them their own culture, which included the language that eventually developed into Sanskrit.

There is no history written in Sanskrit, but from their hymns, *The Vedas*, we know that the Aryans worshipped the forces of nature and that this developed into a system of religious ritual.

In the later *Vedas*, called *Upanishads*, there is a search for the spiritual truth behind the ritual. "What use is the *Rig Veda* to one who does not know the spirit from whom the *Rig Veda* comes." *Upanishad* translates as "to sit next to" and the writings are spiritual discourses from a teacher to his disciples, gathered around him for instruction away from the organized religious system. The first written references to yoga and to meditation are in the *Upanishads*. "When the five senses and the mind are still, and reason itself rests in silence, then begins the path supreme. This calm steadiness of the senses is called yoga."

This teaching is carried further in the *Bhagavad Gita* which was written around 300BC. It is both a spiritual poem and a treatise on yoga set in the epic story of the *Mahabharata*, which tells of the battle between Good and Evil. In the story, the god Krishna tells his devotee Arjuna of the different paths to God, through devotion (*Bhakti* yoga), knowledge (*Jnana* yoga) or action (*Karma* yoga). He also speaks of meditation.

Buddhism

Between the birth of Buddha (around 563BC) and the beginning of the Christian era many religions and philosophies developed. These included orthodox Hinduism (which accepted the teaching of the *Vedas*) and Jainism and Buddhism (rejecting the *Vedas*). All contained elements of yoga within them. The Buddha practiced yoga in the search for enlightenment, finally he rejected both the extremes of personal asceticism and religious ritual and preached "the Middle Way". By the 3rd century BC India was largely Buddhist, but eventually a reformed Hinduism was re-established while Buddhism spread to many other parts of Asia.

Classical yoga and Patanjali's Sutras

Within Hinduism were the six philosophical systems, one of which was yoga. This was not a new teaching, but the result of the long previous development, now written down in eight short, easily-memorized "aphorisms" strung together like beads on a thread (*sutra*). The *Yoga Sutras* written down by Patanjali give a path to be followed by those seeking "the stilling of the mind". Patanjali's aphorisms are precise, practical statements detailing methods of concentrating the mind and the pitfalls of incorrect practice. In the second chapter he gives the eight steps of classical yoga: moral restraints (*yama*), personal discipline (*niyama*), posture (*asana*), breath control (*pranayama*), control of the senses (*pratyahara*), concentration (*dharana*), meditation (*dhyana*) and contemplation (*samadhi*). These steps were meant to complement each other, a disciplined life, posture and steady breathing being essential for the practice of meditation.

Post-classical yoga

Tantrism developed in India from 600–1200AD. This was probably the re-emergence of esoteric teachings that had continued among groups such as the mysterious Vratya brotherhoods that lived on the fringes of society. Tantra incorporated the use of the physical body as a direct instrument for the attainment of spiritual enlightenment. This gave an increased importance to the physical aspect of yoga. In the Hatha yoga writings (from 1000AD) are details of postures (*asanas*) and breathing exercises (*pranayama*) designed to bring health and longevity to the practitioner. Hatha yoga was, however, not merely about the physical exercises: the old texts also stressed the importance of moral discipline and meditation.

Yoga and the Western world

The colonization of India opened up the teaching of yoga to the West. In the 18th century the British Governor-General Warren Hastings encouraged the study of Sanskrit. The *Bhagavad Gita* was translated into English and the *Sacred Books of the East* made available a large number of Sanskrit writings. There were also translations of yoga texts from Chinese into English.

In the late 19th century there was a growing interest in Indian teaching and yoga. Famous Indian teachers like Vivekananda (1863–1902) traveled to Europe and the United States, while Westerners went to India in search of teachers. After the widespread fashion for eastern spirituality, including yoga, in the 1960s, yoga is once more popular in the West for what it can offer both physically and spiritually.

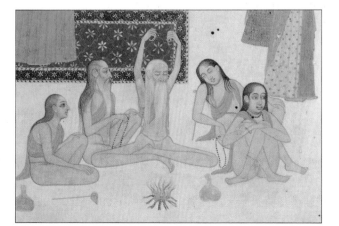

The history of yoga can also be glimpsed in paintings, as in this palace scene (1760).

HEALTHY BODY
H O W   I T   W O R K S

BEFORE YOU START PRACTICING YOGA you need to have an idea of how your body moves and works. Your body's structure is a miraculous balancing act of bones and muscles, which form a framework, and various systems such as breathing, circulation, and digestion.

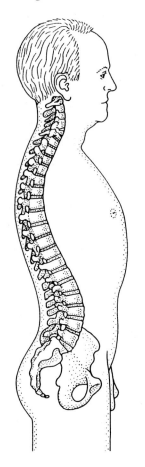

Twenty-four movable vertebrae, the sacrum and coccyx are linked together to form the spine. The spine keeps you upright and protects the spinal cord: the highway of the nervous system. The weight of your body balances on four curves which are found at the back of the neck, the chest, the waist, and the hips.

Spine   The central support of your body is the spine, a string of bony vertebrae with discs of cartilage between them stretching from the base of the skull to the tail bone. These discs are hard on the outside and have a gelatinous nucleus. When the spine is under pressure, for example while standing, water from the center of the disc is squeezed out into the surrounding tissue and the disc becomes flatter. After the pressure is removed the nucleus reabsorbs the water and regains its original thickness. When you get up in the morning you are taller than when you go to bed at night. As you get older the discs lose their ability to re-absorb the water efficiently; they lose depth and you lose height. As the discs flatten the joints at the back of your spine are disturbed, which can lead to osteoarthritis.

The spine is supple enough to move in all directions and strong enough to keep you upright and protect the spinal cord. It is the main pathway of the nervous system. There is only a small amount of movement between the vertebrae but with the overall number of joints, the spine is potentially extremely flexible.

A baby lies curled up inside the womb with its spine still soft and consisting mainly of cartilage in one long curve. After birth the spine forms four curves: the incurve of the neck as the head is lifted up, the curve of the waist as the child starts to crawl and walk, and at the back of your hips and chest your spine stays in the primary outer curves. These four curves balance each other when you are upright and the spine carries the weight of your head and upper body.

The sacrum consists of five vertebrae which fit together to complete the back of the ring of the pelvis. It is like the keystone of an arch and when you stand or sit straight the weight is evenly distributed and the muscles on each side of the body work equally. If you stand or sit with the weight shifted to one side the symmetry of this arch is destroyed and the base of the spine is thrown out of balance.

Yoga stretches and lengthens the spine and improves postural balance. It keeps the spine mobile and the muscles surrounding it strong.

Bones   Some of your bones form three "boxes" which protect the internal organs. The strong flat bones of the skull make a box for the brain. The ribs, breastbone and spine make a flexible cage for the lungs and heart, while the hipbones and sacrum form the pelvis. Good posture occurs when these heavy boxes are balanced one above the other in accordance with the pull of gravity; the four curves of the spine adjusting automatically as you move and the weight supported evenly by each leg in turn.

Bad posture Many things interfere with postural balance, such as slouching in chairs, sitting at desks, driving cars, and many sports. Bad posture can affect all the other systems of the body and your feeling of well-being and energy. Eventually muscles which should contract and lengthen as you move have to stay constantly tight, in order to hold misaligned parts of the body in place, and as a result your natural freedom of movement is restricted.

When the head is carried too far forward your muscles have to work overtime to prevent it dropping even further. This causes kyphosis (round upper back). Lordosis (sway back) happens when the pelvis tilts forward and the curve at the back of the waist is exaggerated. The muscles then have to pull the upper body back in line. Scoliosis occurs when the spine twists sideways in an 'S' bend. Most people have this tendency to a certain degree because of right- or left-handedness but if it is unchecked this will worsen over the years.

Bad posture can develop at any time and many problems that occur in later years are not the inevitable wear and tear of advancing age but the result of thoughtless use of the body.

Joints To keep joints moving freely we need to use their full range. If we fail to do this, in time movement becomes limited and we place strain on adjoining joints. For example, if one hip is stiff it will place strain on the knee of that leg. Sports and exercises which stress the joints can be a contributory factor in the onset of arthritis. Yoga postures, when they are done with an understanding of the body's structure with

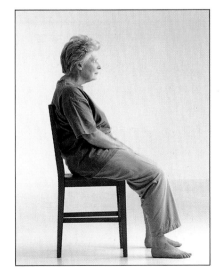

Kyphosis *is caused by carrying your head too far forward. It restricts the movement of the ribcage as you breathe.*

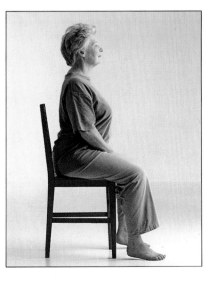

Lordosis *causes low back ache and interferes with the action of the diaphragm.*

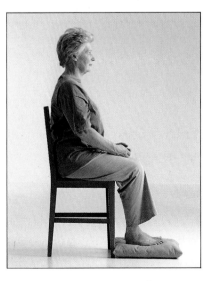

If you sit correctly, *as shown above, there is no unnecessary strain on muscles, ligaments or bones.*

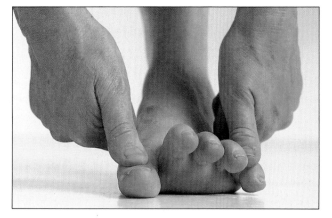

Exercises which maintain the arches of your feet will improve their overall appearance and your posture, balance, and mobility.

breathing and without force, are a restoration of the natural movement and never a distortion of the joint's normal function.

Hips   The hip joints have a ball and socket construction. The ball shape at the top end of the thigh bone fits into the hip socket in the pelvis. They have a large range of movement and bear a great deal of weight. Since the weight of the upper body, head and arms to the legs and feet is transmitted through these joints, they are subject to a great deal of wear and tear.

Today in the West we seldom squat down or sit on the floor and the muscles that surround the hip joints become stiff and tight through lack of use. Eventually these movements become difficult or even impossible. Osteoarthritis of the hip joint is a common complaint of ageing.

Knees   The knee is a hinge which bends and straightens; when your leg is bent there is a little sideways movement. In yoga it is often thought that positions such as Lotus (page 74) require an abnormal movement in the knee, which if attempted by Westerners will very soon cripple them. In fact the movement in Lotus comes from the rotation of the thigh bone in the hip socket

and should put no strain on the knee. Problems arise when people try to put their legs into Lotus before there is enough movement in the hips.

Unlike the elbow, where the shape of the bones prevent it overextending, the back of the knee is held only by ligaments and problems can arise when these are strained. This usually occurs when the weight is incorrectly placed on the balls of the feet so that you push back into the knees. High heels make this worse.

Feet   The 52 small bones of the feet support all your weight, act as shock absorbers as you walk, adapt to uneven surfaces and, if left to their own devices and kept out of shoes, would probably serve you happily to the end of your days. Unfortunately by the time most people reach adulthood feet have had a hard time and are not able to do the job they were designed for.

The foot is constructed like a vault, composed of arch-like structures that should be strong and elastic. There are two arches that run along the length of the foot, one on the outside from the heel to little toe and a deeper one from the heel to the big toe. There are also arches that run across the foot which help to spread the toes. The weight should be borne by the strong bones of the heel with the toes fanning out to help you balance. You can see this natural spreading of the toes in a toddler learning to walk.

The foot can be distorted in any number of ways. Usually the toes become compressed. Sometimes they form an ugly bunion at the base of the big toe, in other cases they curve inward like claws. Both these conditions disturb the working of the arches of the feet, which either collapse and cease to work properly or become stiff and rigid, as well as ugly. If the foot ceases to work properly then all the structures above it are affected. A dropped arch distorts the ankle, which in turn affects the knee and the hip until finally the whole posture is pulled out of line.

Shoulders   These ball and socket joints are the most mobile in the body, but are also where many people accumulate the most tension. Part of this is due to bad carriage of the head and increasing misalignment of the upper spine, which affects the movement of the shoulders. Carrying heavy packages or shoulder-bags, small repeated movements such as typing, driving – in fact, almost all the things you do every day – tend to tighten your shoulders.

Yoga for a healthy body   Yoga *asanas* use the force of gravity from a stable base so that as you breathe out the spine lengthens. The muscles which lie on the front of the spine are released with the relaxation of the diaphragm. As the abdominal muscles become firm at the end of the breath, the curve of the waist extends and the spine lengthens.

Postures evolve from standing, sitting, and lying positions, or even from being on all fours. The base of the position can be the feet, the hands, the elbows or the sitting bones. How far the pose takes you depends on your body type, flexibility, and strength. Learn slowly, using the programs on pages 121–125 as a basis for your practice.

When you do the postures you must work with your body and not against it. Each stretch is a way of freeing your body from stresses and tensions. Yoga allows your natural freedom of movement to be restored and your strength to become regenerated.

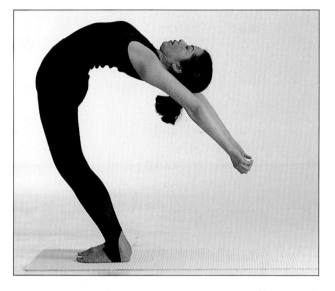

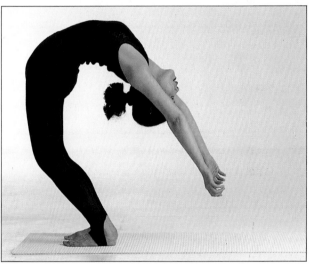

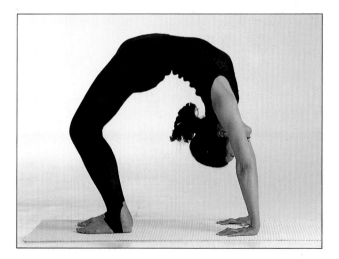

Few people of whatever age are as flexible as this woman in her 50s. She has been practicing yoga for several years.

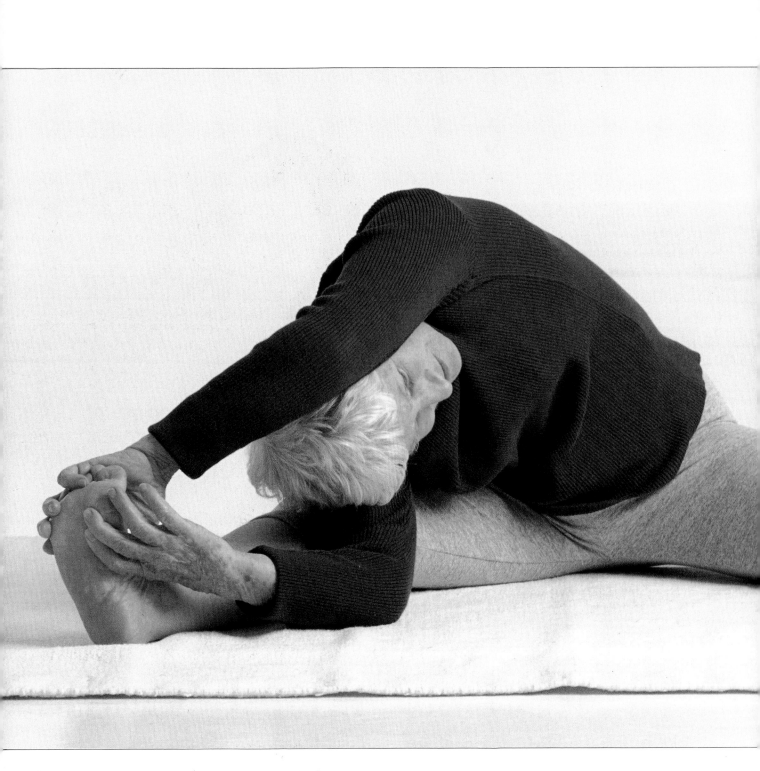

Yoga *asanas* (postures) are the physical strand in the thread of yoga. Their purpose is to adjust and realign your body to bring back its natural balance, by freeing the habitual blocks and tensions acquired over the years. *Asanas* have to be learned slowly so that this can happen gently. It does not matter what age you are or what your state of health is; you can start yoga at any time and practice gentle stretching exercises, relaxation and breathing, even if you are chair-bound.

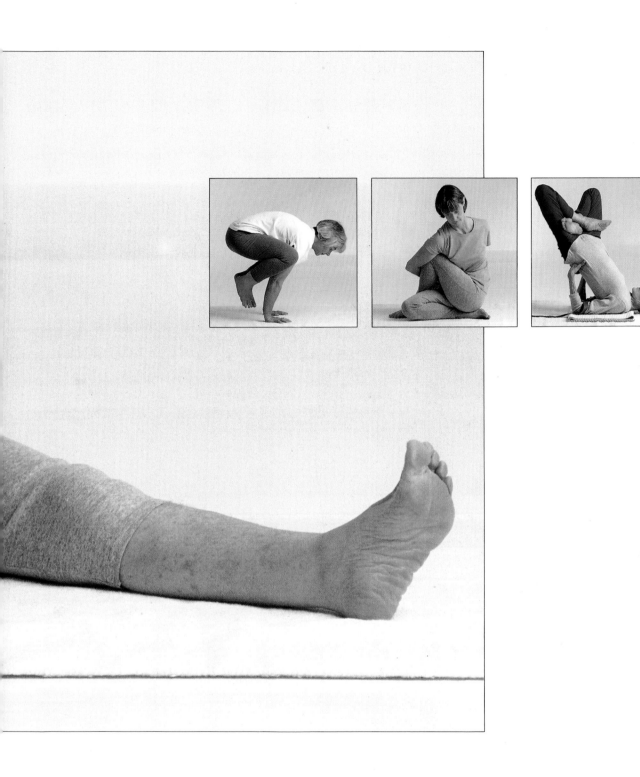

ACTION

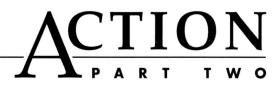

PART TWO

MOUNTAIN and TREE

T A D A S A N A   &   V R K S A S A N A

The idea of a vertical line connecting earth and heaven comes from Vedic times. Later this was symbolized as a mountain, with its roots in the earth and its peak in the heavens. The Mountain is aligned along the pull of gravity and should be both stable and relaxed. Tree pose grows along this same axis with its root going down as the branches stretch upward.

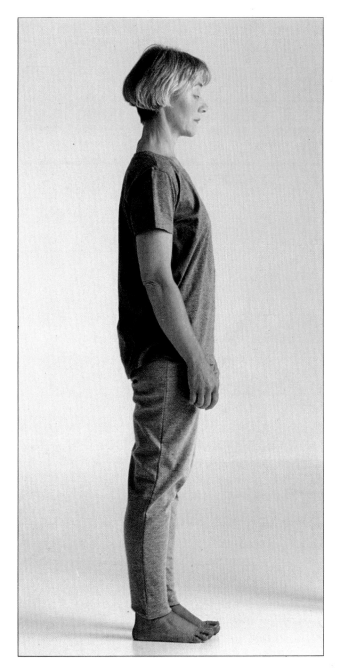

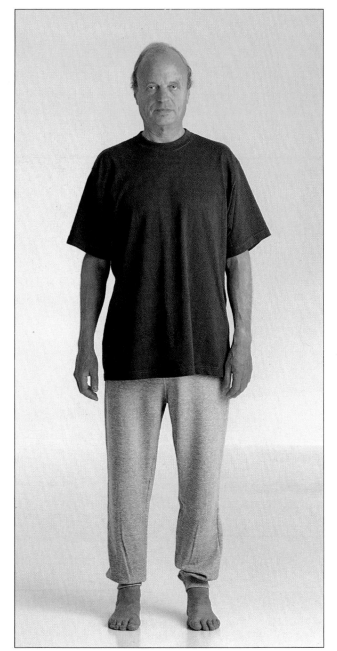

1 *Stand with your feet hip-width apart and parallel, with your weight anchored to the ground through your heels.*

2 *Relax your shoulders and, keeping your knees straight, breathe out and let your spine grow upward.*

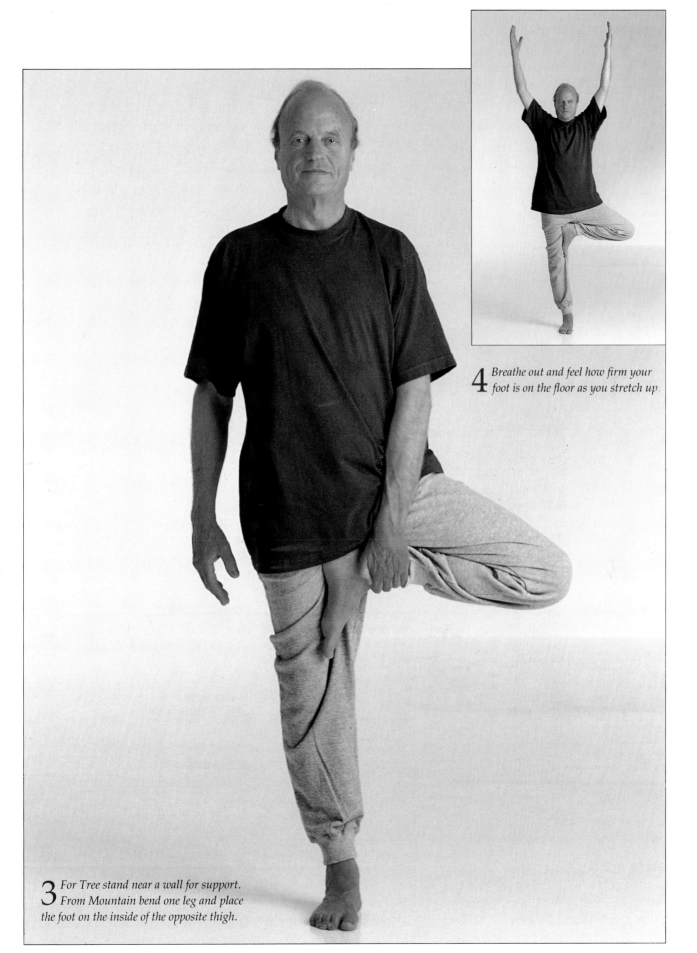

4 *Breathe out and feel how firm your foot is on the floor as you stretch up.*

3 *For Tree stand near a wall for support. From Mountain bend one leg and place the foot on the inside of the opposite thigh.*

STANDING FORWARD BEND
UTTANASANA

In forward bends, the whole of your body from your heels to your head gets longer. You bend from the hips and keep your legs straight and firm. In this pose if you try to touch the floor too soon, when the muscles at the backs of your legs (your hamstrings) are short and tight, you will merely shorten your spine into a curve and strain your lower back. Before starting the pose practice bending forward on to a chair. When your legs and back start to lengthen with your breathing and you become more flexible you will touch the floor easily. Going forward to a chair is also a good way of releasing tension in your shoulders.

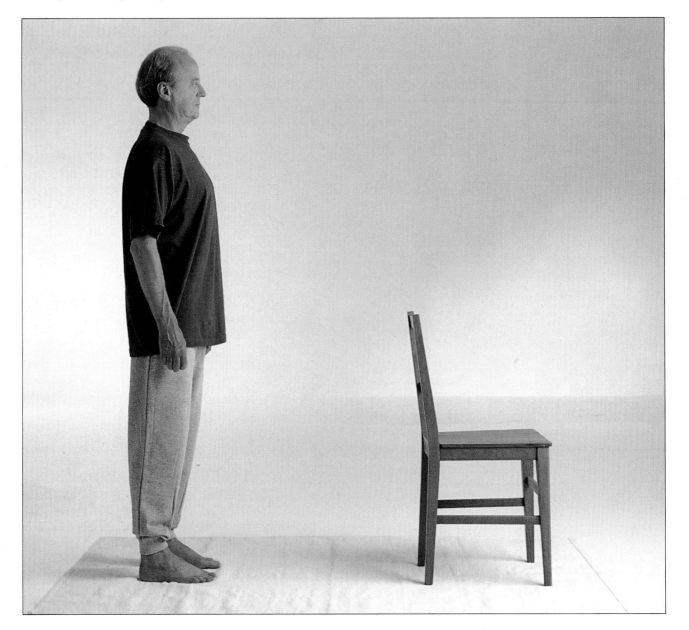

1 *Stand in Mountain (page 18) with a chair in front, keeping all weight on your heels.*

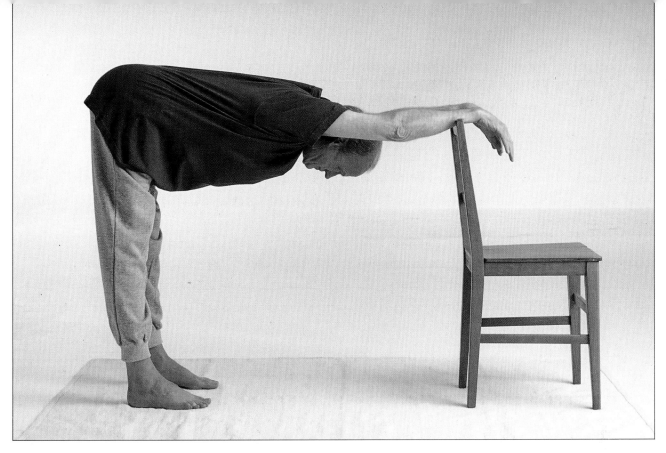

2 *Breathe out and stretch forward to rest your hands on the chair back. Keep hips* *over your heels. Stay for several breaths, lengthening forward on each exhalation.*

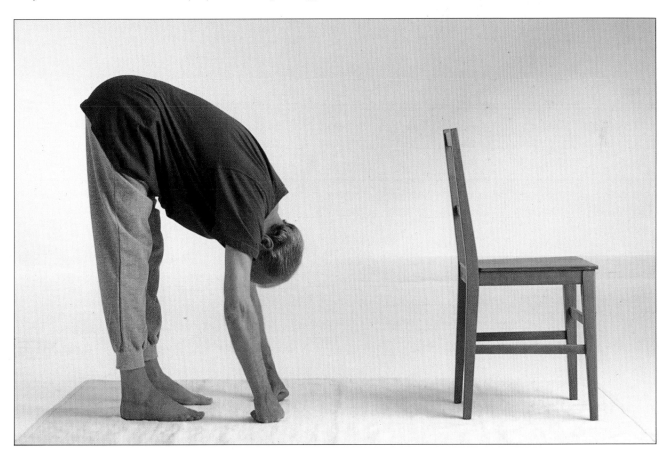

3 *Breathe out again then go down and rest your hands on the floor. Your weight stays* *on your heels. Keep your head, neck and shoulders relaxed during this pose.*

WIDE ANGLE POSE

P R A S A R I T A   P A D O T T A N A S A N A

You can also do a Standing Forward Bend with your legs wide apart and your feet parallel. If you are a beginner, or if you have a problem with balance, stretch forward to a chair, as in the position on page 21, so that your spine can lengthen and the backs of your legs can stretch. Your head will eventually rest on the floor if you lengthen forward but do not force yourself to do this as you will only curve your back. If one hip is stiffer than the other you will tend to be crooked when your legs are apart, so check in a mirror that you are straight as you go forward. Keep your weight on your feet, which should be firmly planted through your heels, as there should be no weight on your hands. When you are steady on your feet you can practice this *asana* with your hands folded up your back with the palms together (see step 3).

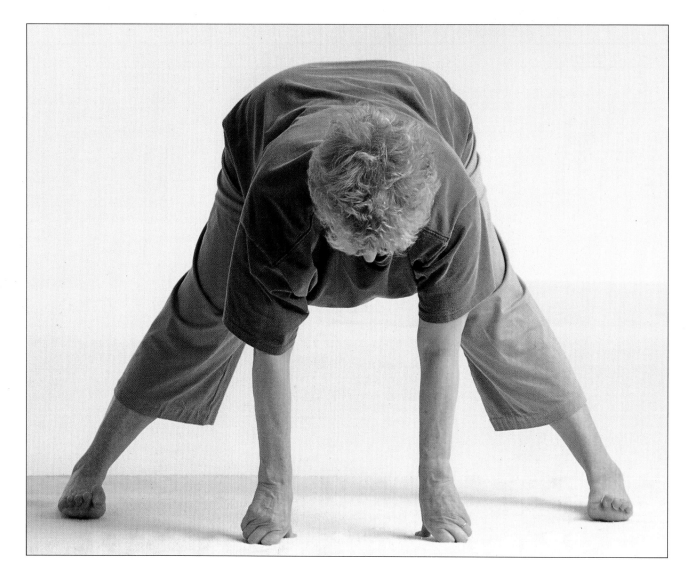

1 *Stand with your legs wide apart and your feet parallel. Breathe out and stretch forward. If your hands do not reach the floor then use a chair (see page 21).*

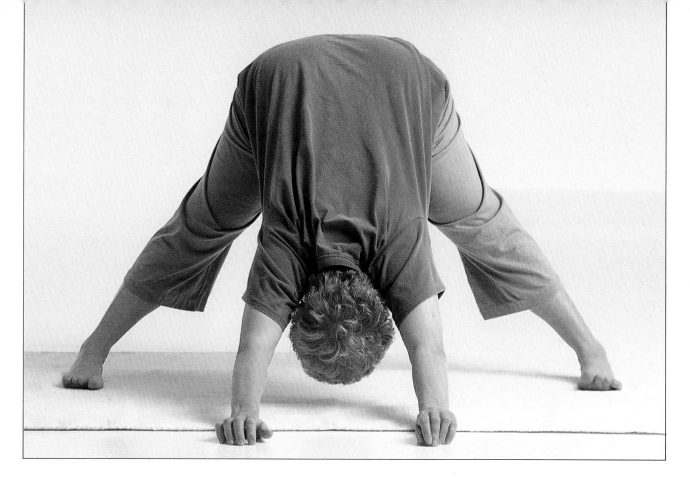

2 *Bend forward, keeping your hips straight.*
Let your spine stretch more on each breath.

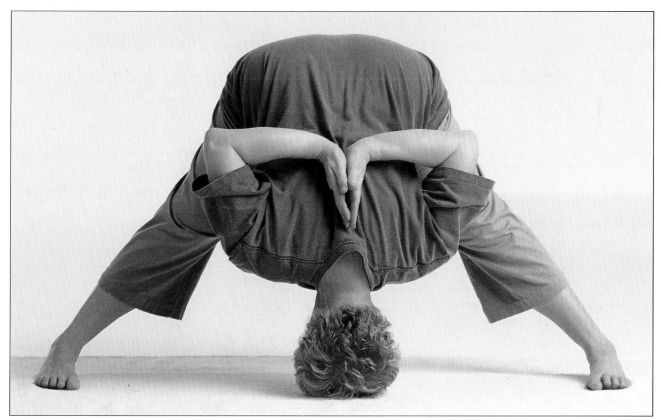

3 *When you are balanced on your heels*
stretch until your head touches the ground.

TRIANGLE FORWARD BEND
PARSVOTTANASANA

The triangle made by your straight legs and the floor forms a strong, stable base from which you can stretch your trunk forward. Your back heel is the anchor which holds your hips steady so that your spine can lengthen. Hands are folded behind your back in the *namaste* position, the traditional greeting in India. Stand straight as in Mountain pose (page 18) then put your palms together behind your back. If this is difficult, hold your elbows behind your back instead.

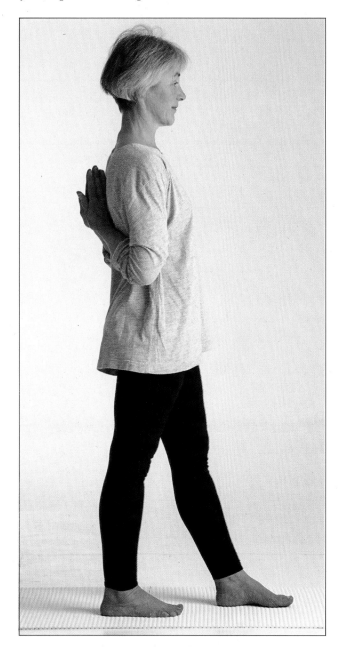

1 *Breathe out and bring your hands up your back, the higher the better. Take one step forward, your weight on your back heel.*

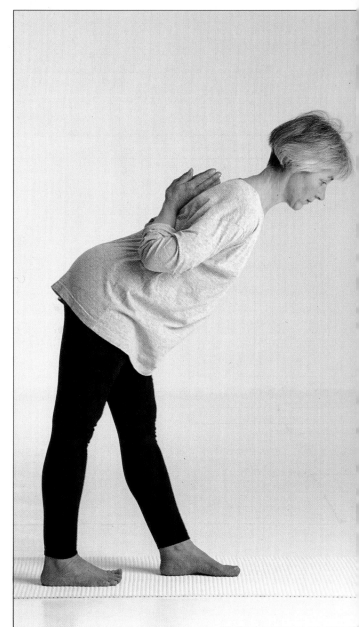

2 *Breathe out and lengthen forward. Don't let your spine collapse into a curve by taking your head too far down your leg.*

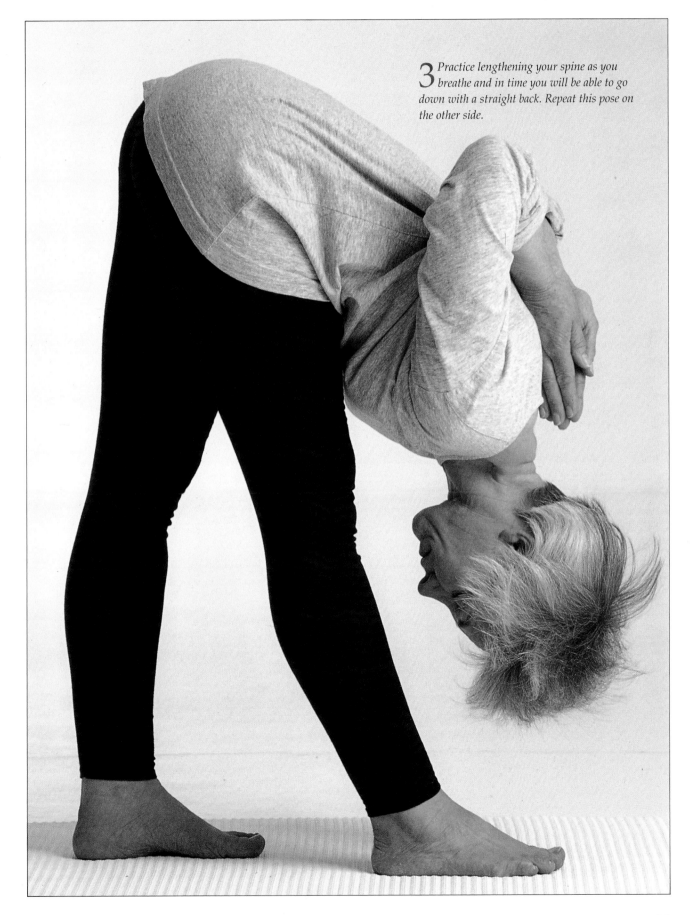

3 *Practice lengthening your spine as you breathe and in time you will be able to go down with a straight back. Repeat this pose on the other side.*

TRIANGLE
TRIKONASANA

In the standing poses your heels anchor your body to the floor so that the spine can lengthen away from the hips. Your shoulders relax so they do not block the action of the upper spine or the breathing. In the Triangle poses both legs remain straight. To stretch further, bend the front leg into Angle Pose (*parsvakonasana*). In all these poses your spine should extend in a straight line. Don't try to go too far as this could make you collapse forwards. For the first few weeks just practice steps 1 and 2. The position starts with Mountain pose (page 18).

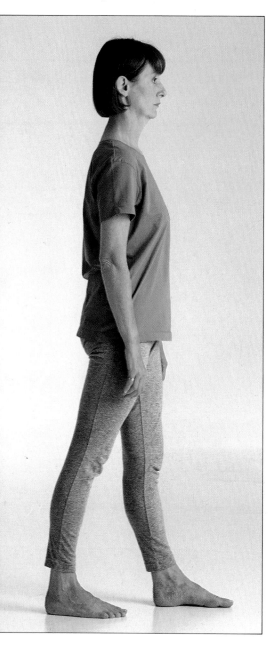

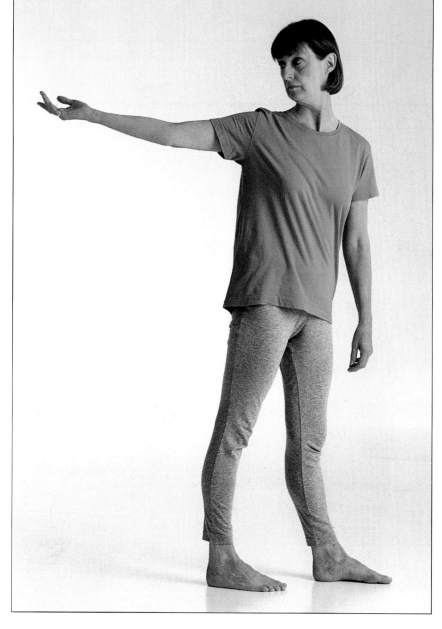

1 *Stand straight, take a step forward, keeping your weight on the back heel.*

2 *Breathe out, turn towards your back foot, extend your arm, then hold the pose.*

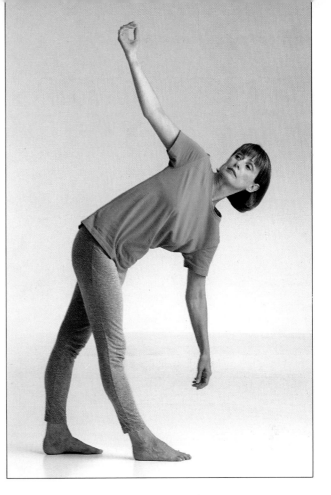

Reverse Triangle (*parivrtta trikonasana*) *The position can be reversed by turning toward your front foot in step 2.*

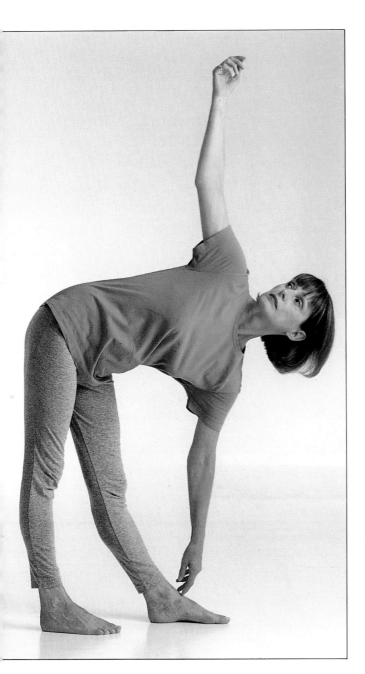

3 *As you breathe out, extend your spine sideways, stretching your arm up and keeping all your weight on your back heel. Come up and repeat on the other side.*

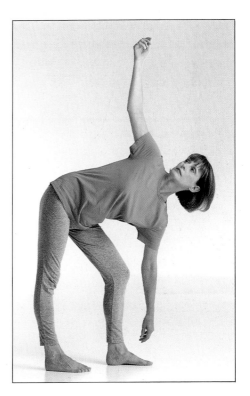

Angle Pose *From step 2 bend your front knee, keeping all the weight on your back foot.*

HALF-LOTUS STANDING
ARDHA PADMA PADOTTANASANA

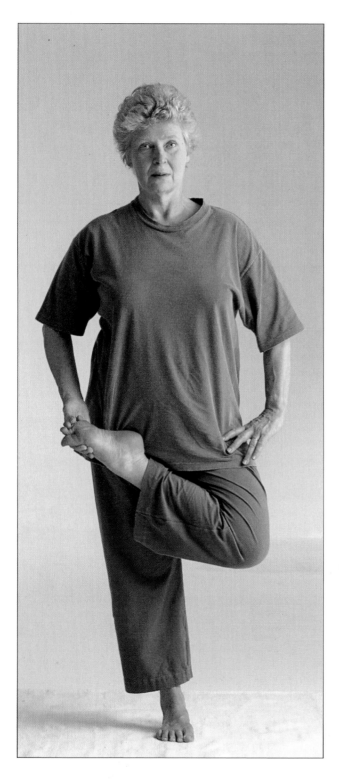

In Lotus (page 74) your thigh has to turn out at the hip and your spine extend away from the pelvis. When you stand you can use the force of gravity to help release the hip so that the thigh can drop down as it turns out. If you find it difficult, support your knee on a chair as you breathe out and let the hip relax. When the foot is in Lotus position it rests in the groin and as you bend forward it helps to keep the front thigh muscles of the straight leg passive.

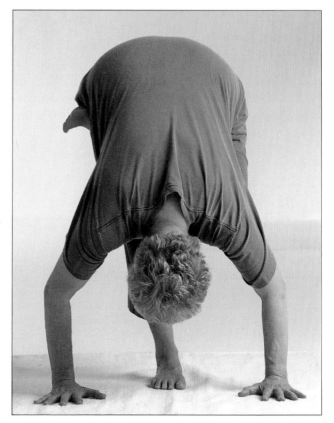

1 *Stand on one leg and take the other into Half-Lotus pose, letting the knee drop down toward the floor as the foot comes up.*

2 *When the Lotus foot is high in the groin breathe out and bend forward, keeping the bent knee pointing toward the ground.*

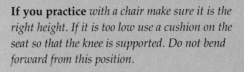

If you practice *with a chair make sure it is the right height. If it is too low use a cushion on the seat so that the knee is supported. Do not bend forward from this position.*

STANDING TWIST

PARIVRTTA PARSVAKONASANA 1

This twisting movement toward your bent leg is
the foundation for all the other twisting *asanas*.
Angle Pose Twist (page 38), Sage Twist (page 96)
and Half-Sage Twist (page 98) all stem from this
straight, stable position where your spine
lengthens as it turns. It is much easier to learn to
extend your spine with the exhalation from a
standing position than it is when you are sitting
down, particularly if you are stiff in the hips.
The vertical line of Mountain (page 18) must be
maintained throughout this twist. Your hips
must stay facing the chair as your upper body
turns until your shoulders are parallel with your
bent thigh. If you have a problem with balance,
stand near a wall, or first practice the Chair
Twist on page 41.

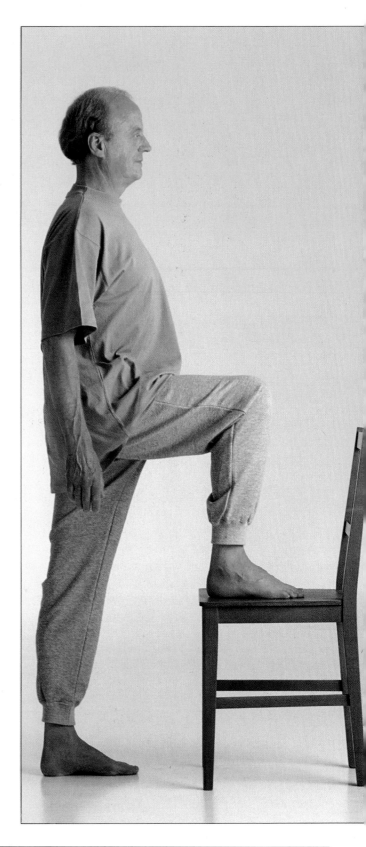

1 *Stand in Mountain (page 18) and place one
foot on the seat of a chair in front of you.
Keep your weight on the heel of your standing
leg and lengthen upward as you breathe out.*

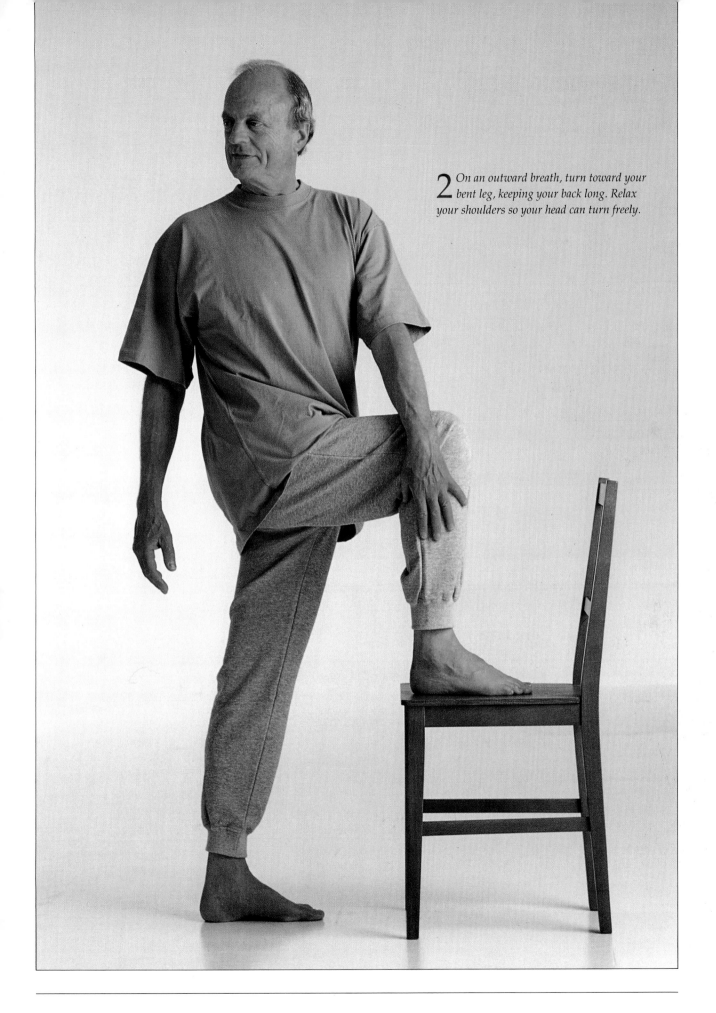

2 *On an outward breath, turn toward your bent leg, keeping your back long. Relax your shoulders so your head can turn freely.*

WARRIOR
VIRABHADRASANA

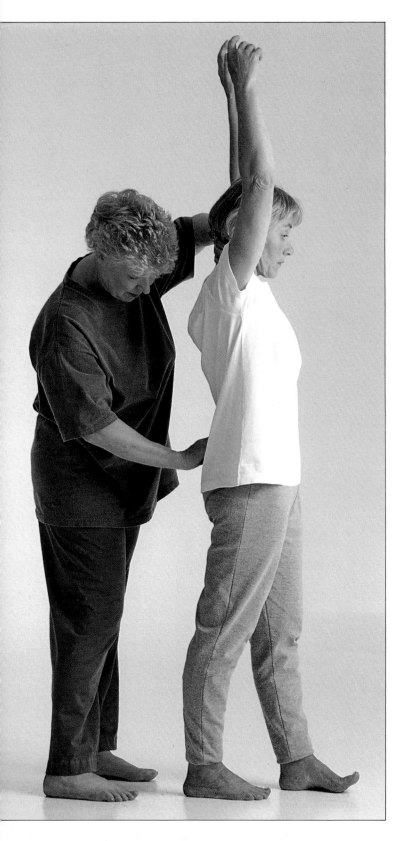

This pose is named after a mythical warrior who rose from the ground to wreak vengeance on a demon. It is a strong, powerful balance that extends breath by breath from a stable base.
The spine lengthens as the raised leg is stretched away from the trunk. The knee of the raised leg faces the floor and the back of the pelvis should be facing the ceiling. There is a straight line from the hands to the raised foot throughout.
The pose should not freeze or become blocked. Stand in Mountain pose (page 18) to begin.

1 *Take one step forward. Breathe out and raise your arms, lengthening upward.*

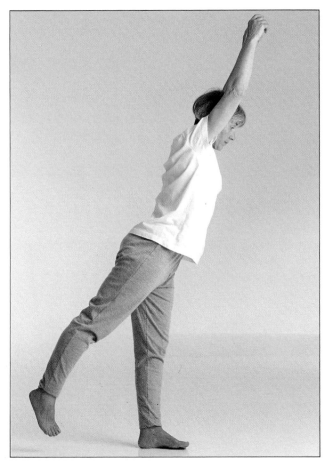

2 *Transfer your weight on to your front foot, letting your back leg lift up.*

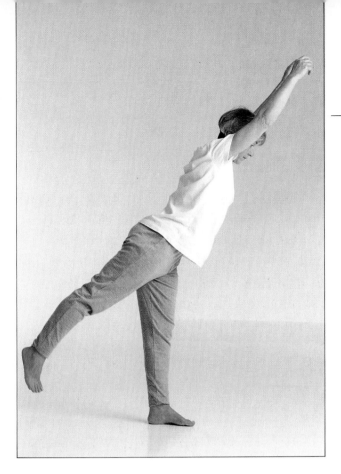

3 *Stretch your leg away from your trunk and lengthen forward and up on the exhalation.*

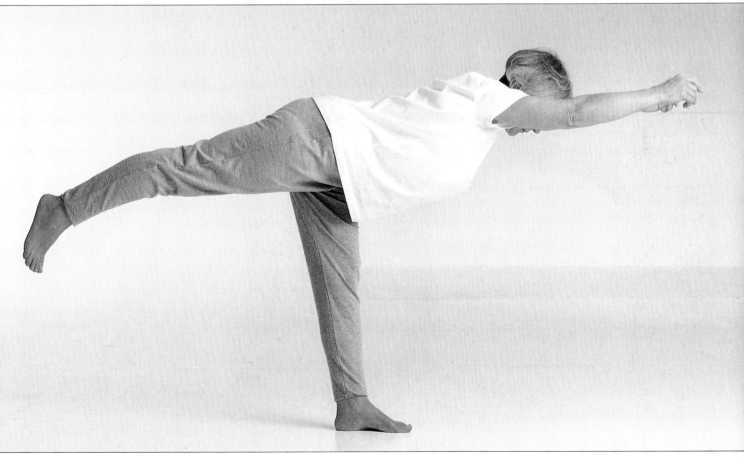

4 *Eventually your raised leg, trunk and arms become horizontal. The back of your waist* *and neck should continue to extend as you go further into the pose.*

HALF-MOON

ARDHA CHANDRASANA

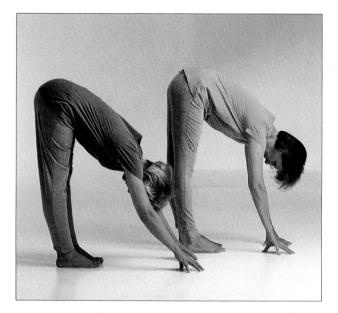

Before you attempt this graceful pose you must be able to do the Standing Forward Bend (page 20) with both your hands touching the floor. The raised leg stretches away from your hips and allows the spine to extend toward your head, giving a wonderful sense of freedom. You need a good sense of alignment for this pose, which brings balance and concentration.

1 *Stand in Mountain pose (page 18), breathe out and bend forward putting both hands on the floor a little way in front of you.*

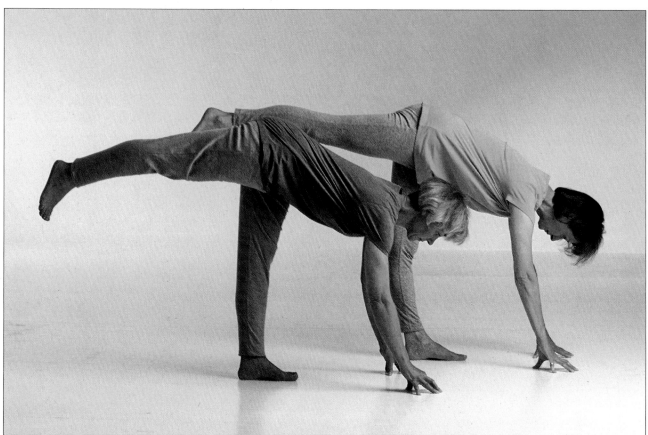

2 *Hold step 1 for a few breaths, letting your back lengthen as the weight stays on your heels. Then breathe out and raise your right leg,* *stretching it away from your trunk, which will lengthen forward toward your head. Your body must be well aligned for you to balance.*

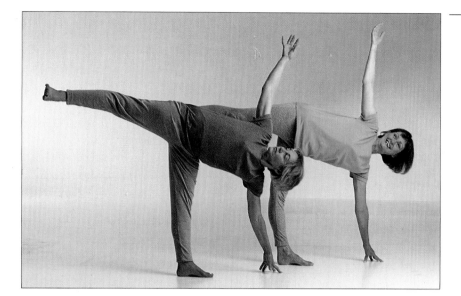

3 Take your right hand off the floor. As your right leg stretches, with every breath let your whole body and raised leg turn so that you are facing forward with your arms in a vertical line. Repeat the pose on the other side.

Half-Moon Twist *This pose can also be done as a twist by turning away from your raised leg and raising the opposite arm.*

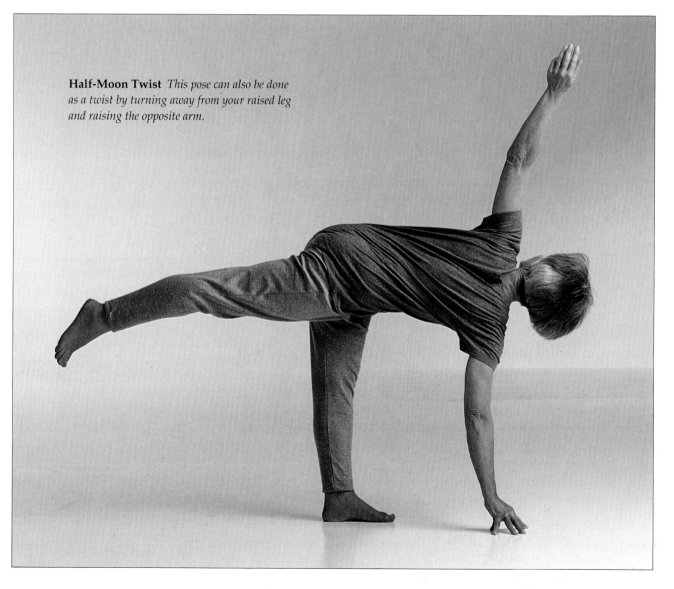

CRANE

BAKASANA

This compact, bird-like pose balances on your hands which are the feet of the bird and the roots of the position. As you come into the pose your wrists have to go down into the ground as you lift up and forward. This requires concentration and coordination rather than muscular effort. It is a position that centers you and brings a great feeling of inner strength once you have mastered it. As you transfer your weight to your hands, your feet will lift off the floor. Put a cushion in front of you if you are worried about toppling over on to your face.

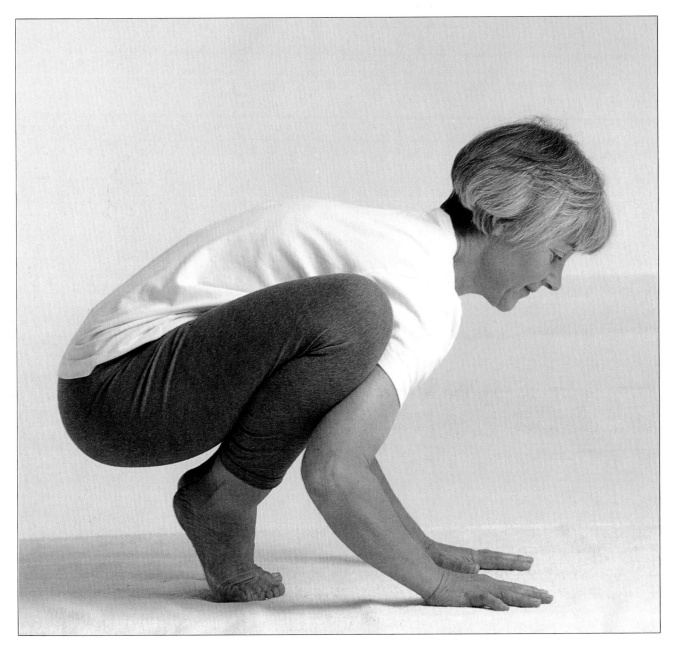

1 *Squat, bringing arms inside your knees and placing hands on the floor in front of you.*

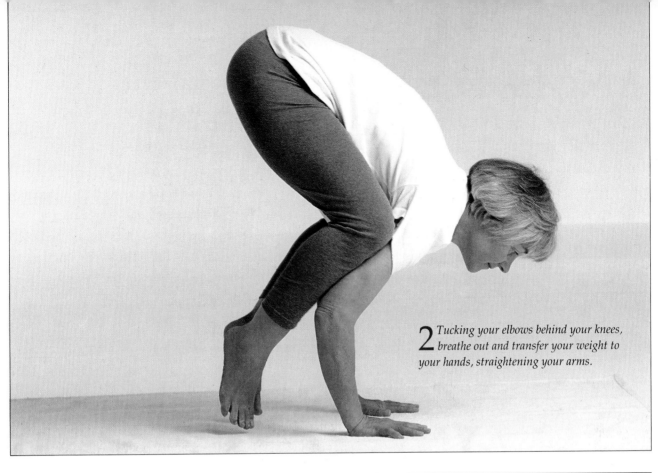

2 *Tucking your elbows behind your knees, breathe out and transfer your weight to your hands, straightening your arms.*

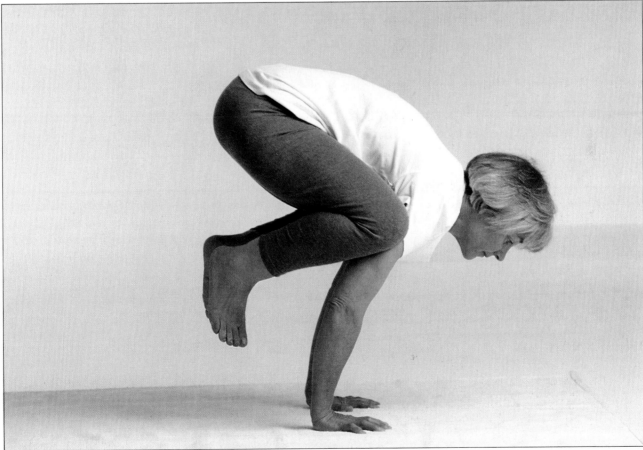

3 *Lift your feet off the floor as you come up and take your elbows over your wrists.*

ANGLE POSE TWIST

PARIVRTTA PARSVAKONASANA 2

This *asana* is a twist variation of step 4 in the Salute to the Sun (page 102). Step 1 of this pose is a kneeling version of the Standing Twist (page 30), which you should learn before trying this more intense stretch. It may take some time for you to bring your hands together behind your back in step 3. If so, stay in step 2, letting your spine grow longer as you relax and turn further into the pose. Don't push against your leg with your elbow or tighten your shoulders. The bent upper knee in this twist should be kept at a right angle with your heel down on the floor.

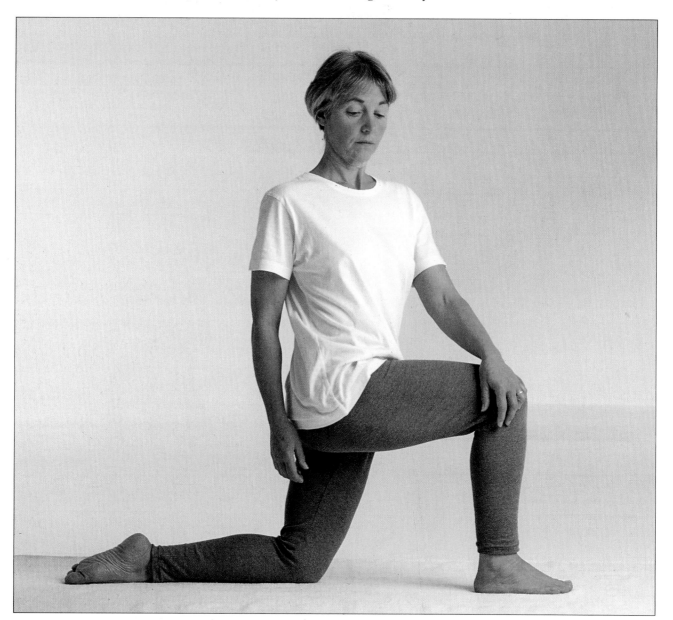

1 *Go down on one knee with the other leg bent in front of you. Lengthen as you breathe out and turn toward your upper leg.*

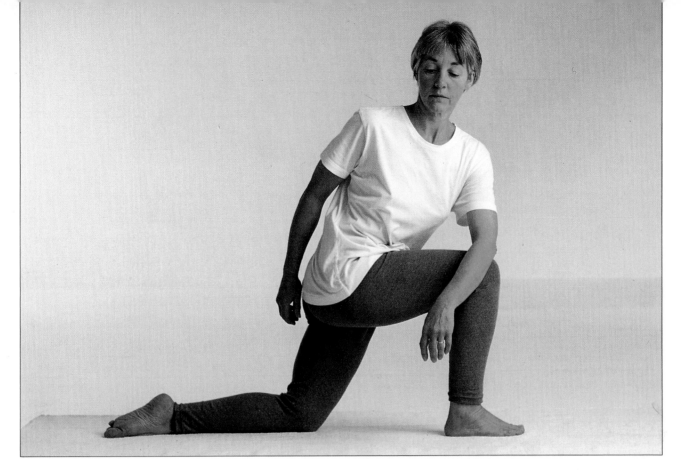

2 *Lean forward as you breathe out.*
Drop your arm outside your front knee.

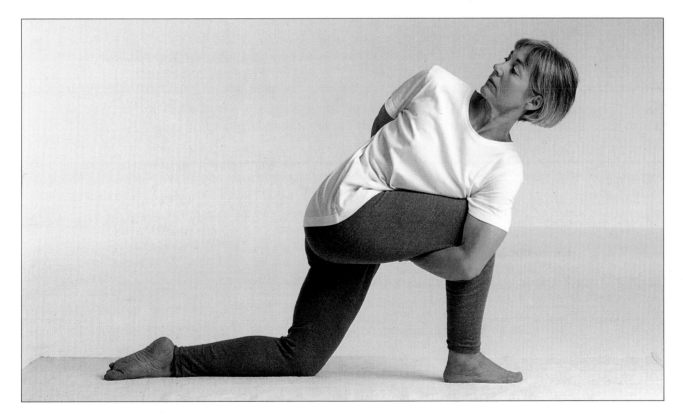

3 *When the back of your armpit is close to*
your knee you should easily be able to bend
your elbow and hold hands behind your back.

CHAIR POSES

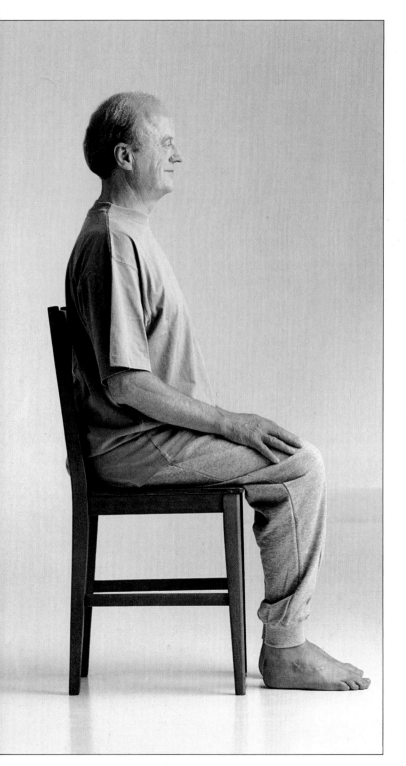

If you are unsteady on your feet some yoga stretches can be done from a chair. The principle of breathing as you straighten your spine to go into the positions is an effective way to improve posture and well-being, whether you are standing, sitting or lying down. You need to move to stay healthy even if you are chair-bound. Sitting well with your hips down and your back straight means that your heart, lungs and internal organs can work more efficiently. The forward stretches shown on pages 42–43 can also be done with your legs wide apart.

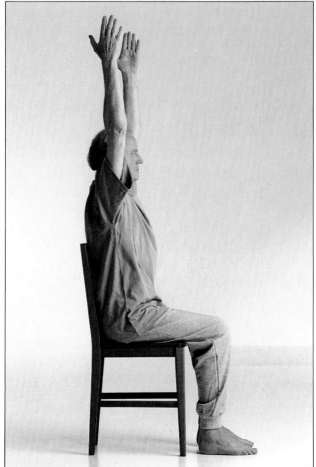

1 *Sit up straight so that your lower back touches the back of the chair. Draw in your abdomen as you breathe out and sit up tall.*

2 *Raise your arms as you breathe out, keeping your hips down and your lower back touching the chair.*

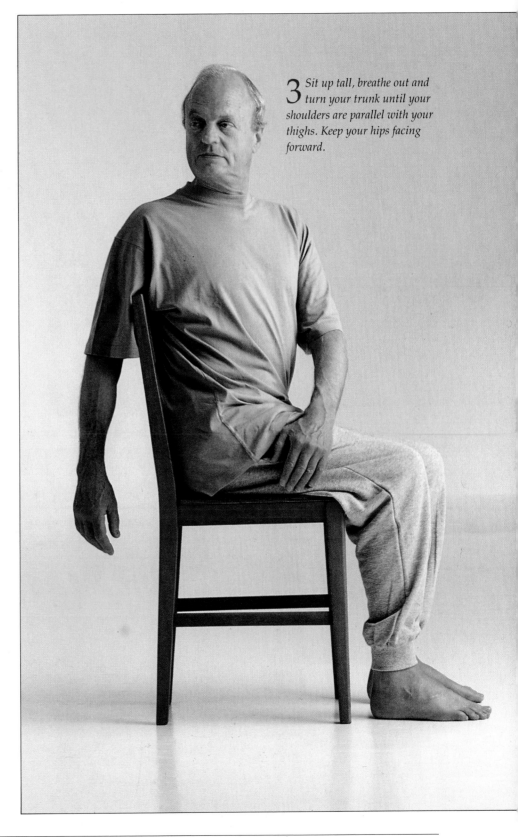

3 *Sit up tall, breathe out and turn your trunk until your shoulders are parallel with your thighs. Keep your hips facing forward.*

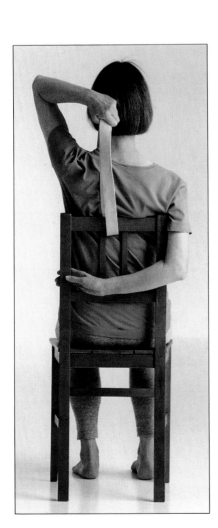

4 *Hold the back of the chair with one arm. Raise your other arm to hold a belt looped over the back of the chair.*

If you have short legs *you will need to put a cushion or a book under your feet so they can rest firmly on the floor. You can use this straight pose for breathing and meditation.*

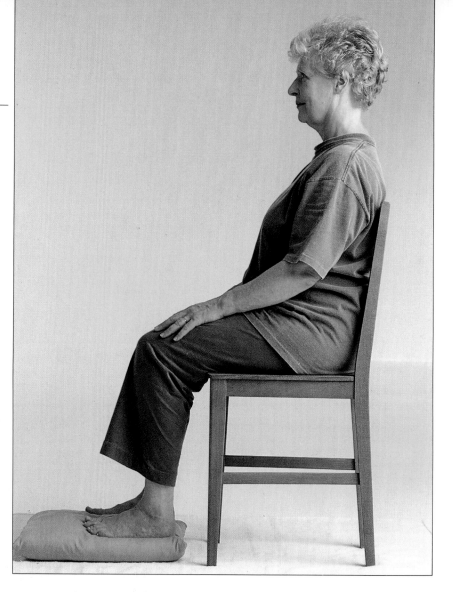

From the straight sitting position *you can lengthen your spine forward by bending to rest your hands on a chair in front of you.*

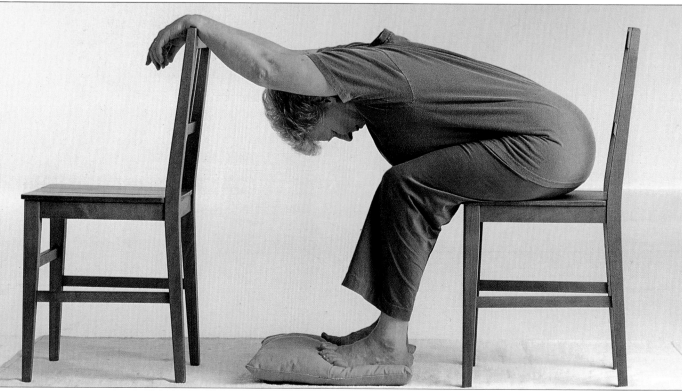

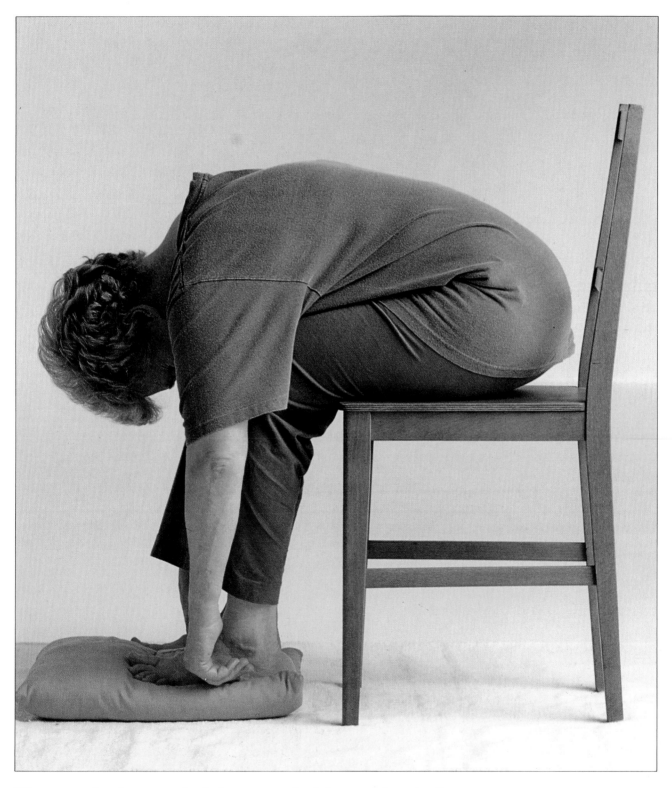

When you can lengthen your spine *in the forward stretch you can bend further by taking* *your hands down toward your feet. Keep your hips firmly down as you do this.*

SHOULDER STAND
SARVANGASANA

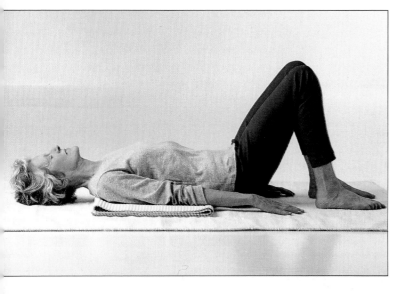

Shoulder Stand is learned before Headstand (page 50). If you learn to keep your weight on your elbows and go up without tightening your shoulders and compressing your neck, it is a calming pose. Your neck must be straight, so it is important to take time in step 1 to feel if you are lying symmetrically. Do not attempt to straighten your head when you are upside down but come down and start again. If this exercise is difficult try resting your feet against a wall (*see opposite*). Take medical advice before doing inverted poses if you have any physical problems affecting your heart, neck, blood pressure or your eyes.

1 *Lie on your back with your shoulders and arms on a blanket. Keep your palms down.*

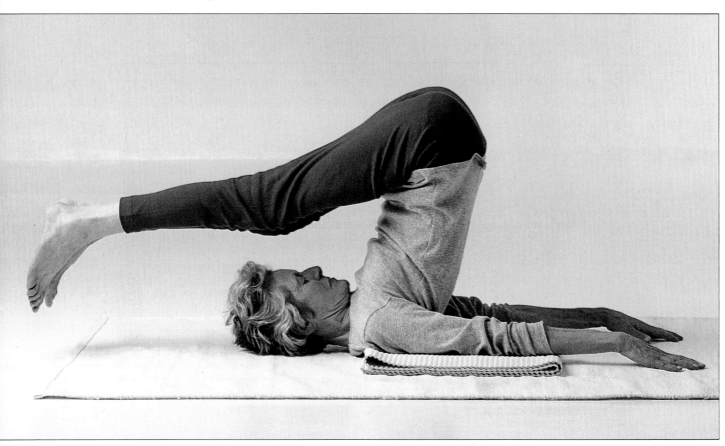

2 *Breathe out, keeping your elbows down.*
Lift up and bring your hips over your head.

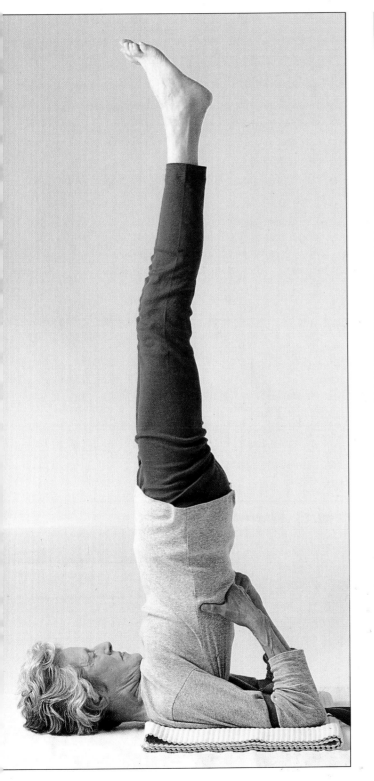

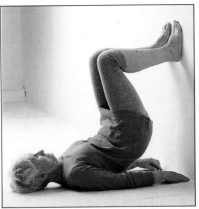

If Shoulder Stand is difficult *lift your hips by pushing your feet against a wall.*

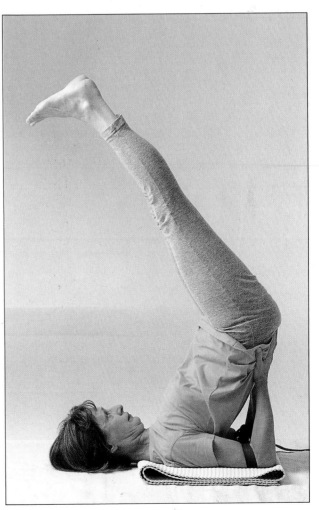

3 *Support your back with your hands and lift up vertically, using a belt if necessary.*

If you find it hard to come up *keep your weight on your elbows and take your time.*

MORE SHOULDER STANDS
SARVANGASANA

When you are steady in Shoulder Stand and can extend without tensing your neck and shoulders, try these stretches for the legs and hips. The roots of the Shoulder Stand must be stable and the spine should continue to lengthen as you do these stretches. The position with straight legs is an excellent exercise for strengthening injured knees as it stretches the upper legs strongly. It is also helpful if you suffer from varicose veins. The poses with the legs in Lotus are more difficult and should not be tried unless you can do Lotus easily (page 74). If you are steady in Shoulder Stand you can use one hand at a time to put your legs into Lotus.

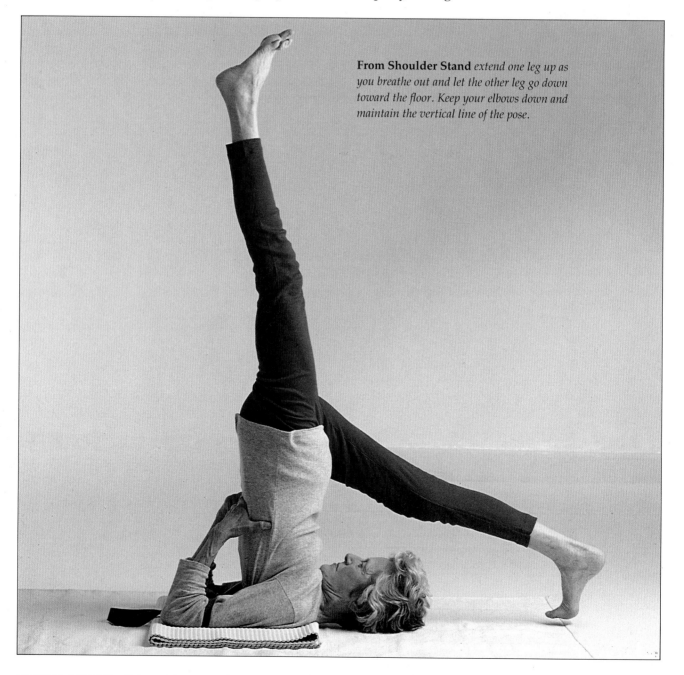

From Shoulder Stand *extend one leg up as you breathe out and let the other leg go down toward the floor. Keep your elbows down and maintain the vertical line of the pose.*

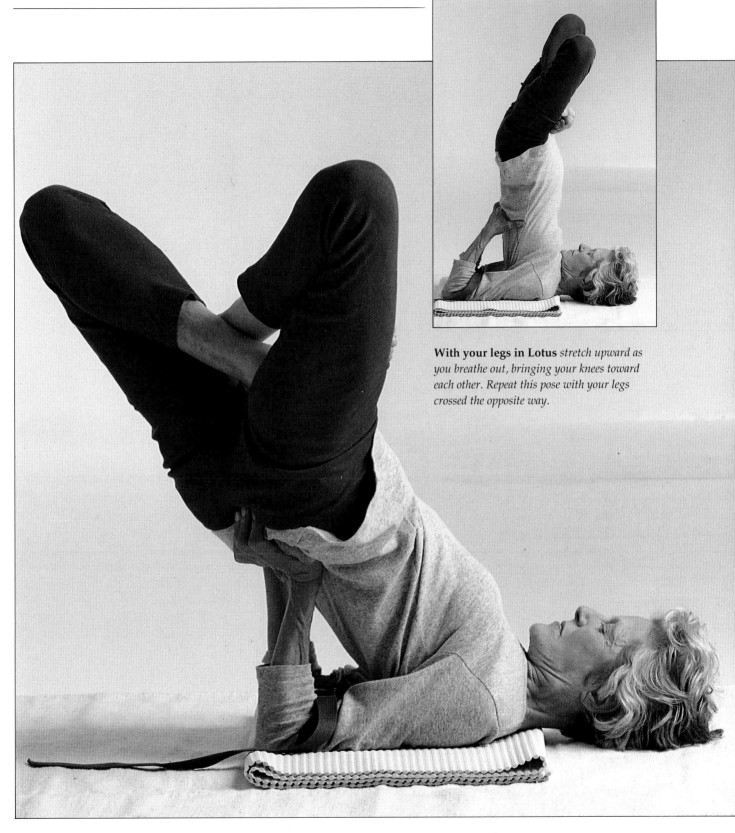

With your legs in Lotus *stretch upward as you breathe out, bringing your knees toward each other. Repeat this pose with your legs crossed the opposite way.*

Turn your trunk *to the left, placing your hands under your pelvis. Extend your knees* *away from you. Repeat on the other side, then do with your legs crossed the other way.*

PLOW

H A L A S A N A

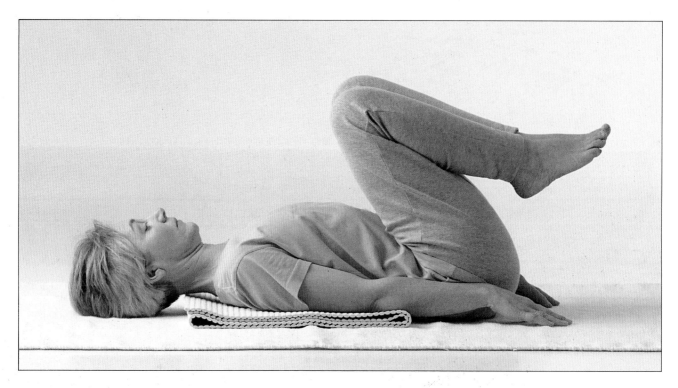

1 *Lie with a blanket under your shoulders and elbows. Rest your arms, palms down.*

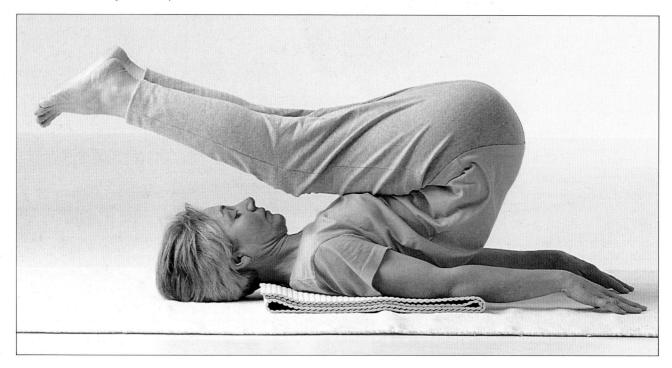

2 *Keeping your arms down, breathe out and let your hips roll up over your head.*

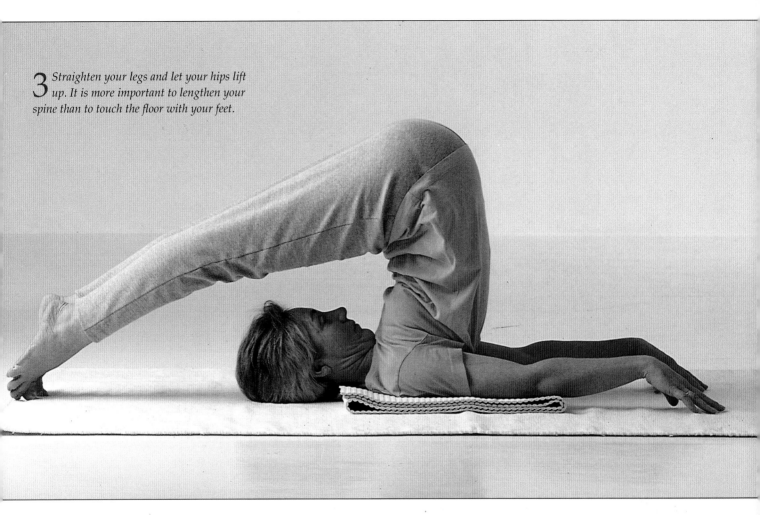

3 *Straighten your legs and let your hips lift up. It is more important to lengthen your spine than to touch the floor with your feet.*

Plow is one of the Shoulder Stand cycle of *asanas*. As in Shoulder Stand you should keep your weight on your elbows and avoid tightening your shoulders or tensing your neck. Also, make sure you are lying straight before you go up into position. You can practice it as a continuation of Shoulder Stand by dropping your legs down as you breathe out after a few minutes in the pose.

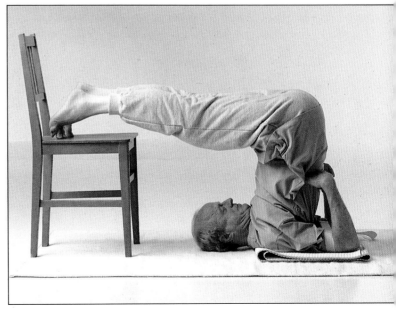

If Plow is difficult, *use a chair and support your back with your hands.*

HEADSTAND
SIRSASANA

Inverted poses are particularly associated with yoga. Headstand is the "king" of the *asanas*. From a stable base your body stretches upward, balancing with the pull of gravity at each breath. It is a strong, powerful pose that should never be tense or rigid. In practice, it is always followed by Shoulder Stand (page 44), "queen" of the *asanas*, which has to be perfected before you attempt Headstand. In inverted poses there is a tendency to tighten your shoulders and tense your neck to push yourself up into the position. This makes the base of the pose unstable and compresses the vertebrae in the neck, so you must spend time on the preparatory stages of the pose before lifting your feet off the floor. If you have neck problems this position can be dangerous. Seek the help of a qualified teacher if you have postural misalignments or arthritis.

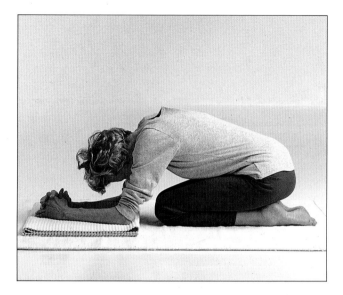

1 *Sit on your heels then rest your elbows on a folded blanket in front of you. Stretch your arms until your hands meet. Loosely clasp your fingers, turning your wrists inward.*

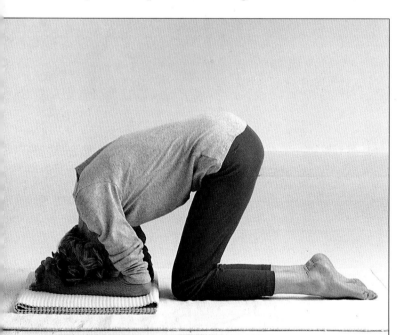

2 *Breathe out. Rest the crown of your head on the blanket inside the triangle made by your elbows and wrists. The back of your neck should lengthen. Hold position for a few breaths.*

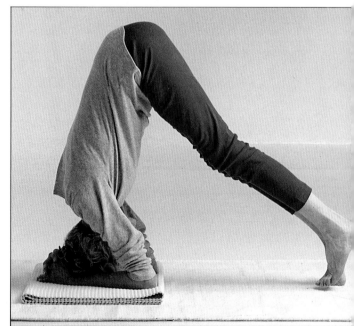

3 *Breathe out. Straighten your legs to raise your hips, keeping the weight on your elbows. The back of your body should lengthen from the back of your head to your hips.*

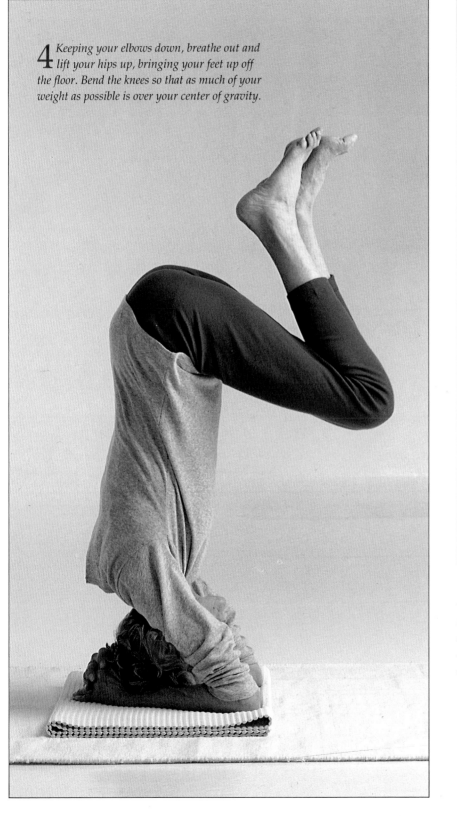

4 *Keeping your elbows down, breathe out and lift your hips up, bringing your feet up off the floor. Bend the knees so that as much of your weight as possible is over your center of gravity.*

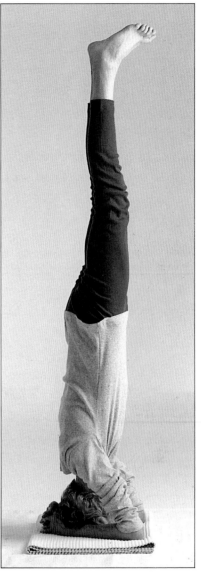

5 *Straighten your legs as you breathe out. Let your abdomen come in and the back of your waist extend. Stretch the back of your legs so that there is a straight line from your shoulders through your hips and knees to your ankles.*

MORE HEADSTANDS
SIRSASANA

When Headstand is completely stable with your elbows rooted to the ground, the body balances freely with the spine extending in its four curves as you breathe. You can stretch the legs and hips further as in this position they have no weight to bear. In all these positions your elbows must stay down on the floor so that your neck remains long and there is no tension in your shoulders. This lets your spine lengthen upward.

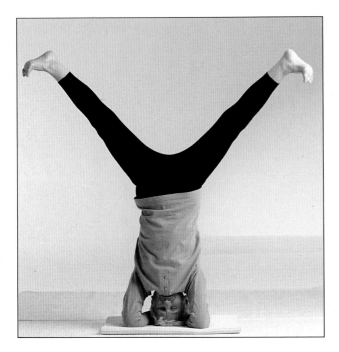

From Headstand *breathe out, stretch up and open your legs wide. Keep your knees straight and make sure you take them down evenly.*

You can also get *a good stretch in your hips and lower back by doing Lotus while you are in Headstand. You need to be able to put your legs into position without using your hands.*

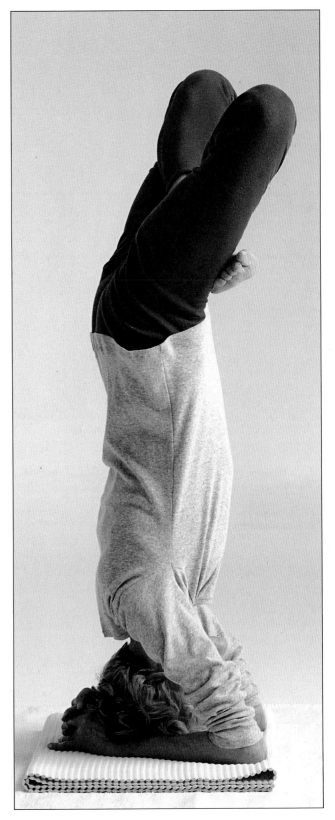

Taking one leg down *in Headstand enables you to lengthen the other side upward strongly, stretching the back of your leg to lift the pelvis. This is an excellent position for injured knees.*

When the base of the pose *is really stable you can extend the spine backward. This full extension of the spine is for the very few who can keep their weight on their elbows as they drop back.*

LEG STRETCHES
SUPTA PADANGUSTHASANA

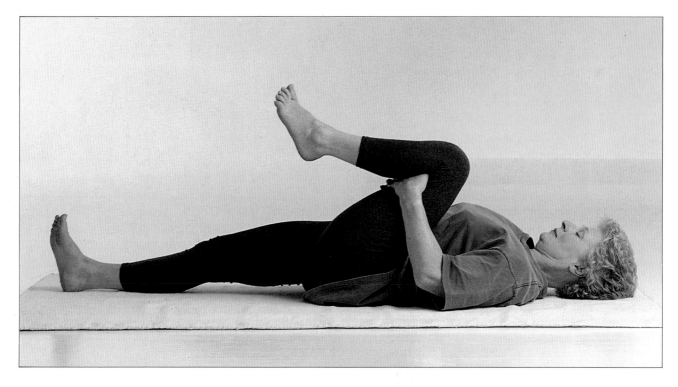

1 *Hold one leg behind your thigh, breathe out and stretch your other leg away from you.*

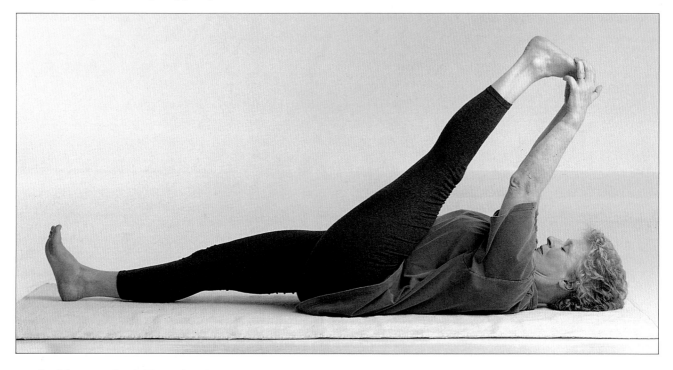

2 *Straighten your leg, hold your foot then stretch the other leg as you breathe out.*

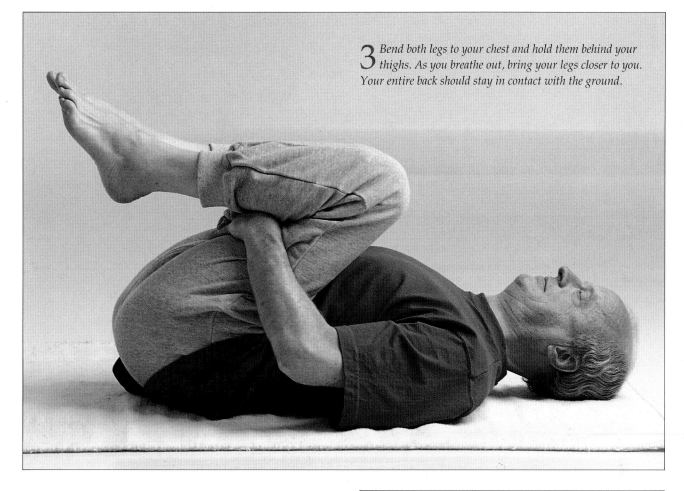

3 *Bend both legs to your chest and hold them behind your thighs. As you breathe out, bring your legs closer to you. Your entire back should stay in contact with the ground.*

When you lie on your back your legs do not bear any weight and it is much easier to exercise stiff hip joints. These leg stretches are particularly effective if practiced after you have been upside down in Headstand (page 50) and Shoulder Stand (page 44). They are also a good way of warming up at the start of your practice. If your chin tips upward and your neck shortens because your upper back is stiff, put a small pillow under your head while you do these exercises. Use a belt if it makes this *asana* easier.

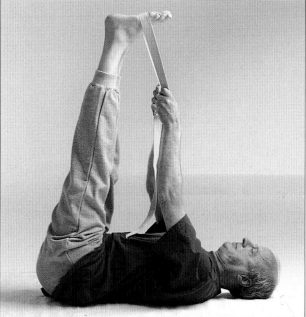

4 *Straighten your legs while breathing out. Bring your feet to your head.*

FLOOR TWIST

JATHARA PARIVARTANASANA

Lower back ache can be relieved by this simple supine twist, which rotates the spine while you are fully supported by the floor. If your head tips backward because your upper back is rounded and your shoulders are stiff, put a small pillow under your head to allow your neck to stretch. This is also a good exercise to do if you find it difficult to sleep as it releases the tension in your shoulders and neck which comes from tossing and turning in bed. Keep your spine as flat on the floor as possible.

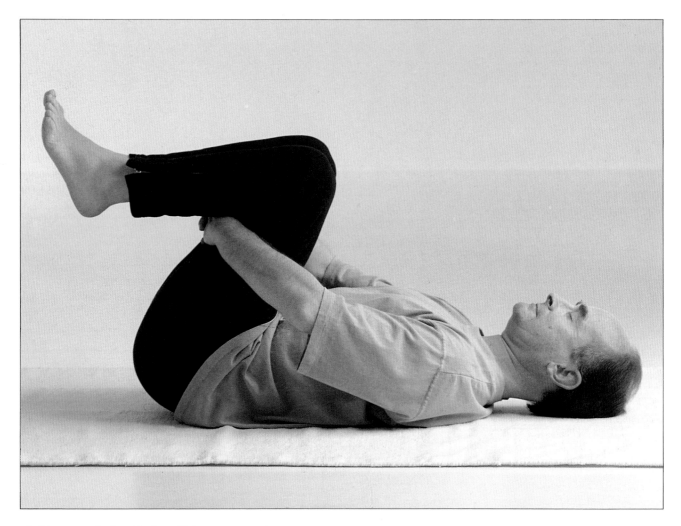

1 *Lie on your back on the floor. Hug your knees, holding them behind your thighs.*

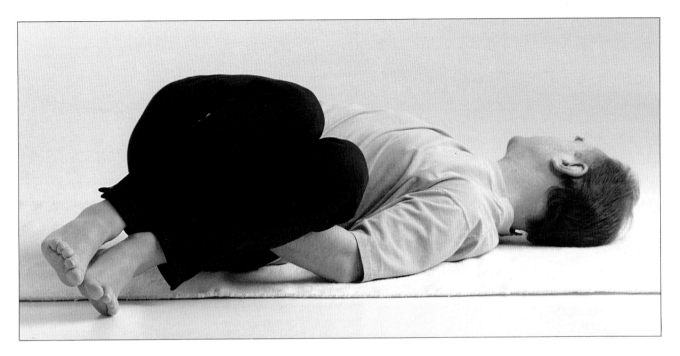

2 Breathe out, rolling your head to the right.
Roll your hips to the left on the next breath.

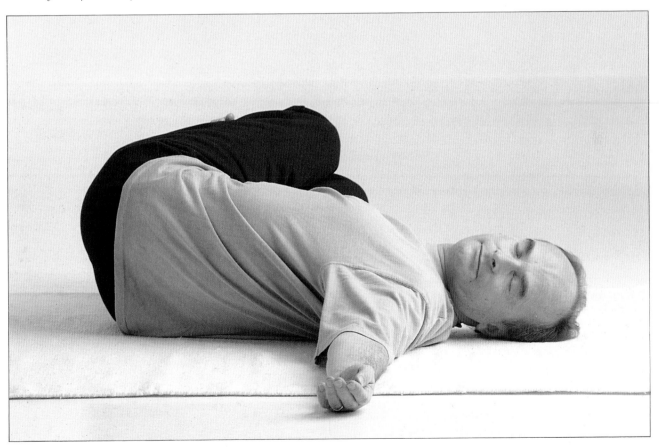

3 Stay for several breaths and let your
abdomen draw inward as you breathe out
so that your lower back lengthens. Then come back to
the center and repeat on the other side.

FLOOR POSES

These simple stretches can be practiced as a preliminary warm-up for your yoga practice. They can also be part of a simple routine for the less mobile, or as a relaxation after a hard day when you have been standing a lot. They are excellent if you suffer from varicose veins or swollen ankles. Make sure you are lying straight with your hips close to the wall before you start. If your upper back and shoulders are stiff and your head tips backward, you will need a small pillow under your head to keep your neck relaxed. The best place to do these exercises is on the floor, as you need a hard flat surface beneath you. However you can do them lying on a firm bed with your legs stretched up the wall, but be careful you don't fall off. Practice these stretches in the order shown here. You can then practice the preparation for Shoulder Stand (page 44) and the Floor Twist (page 56) if you wish. Stay in these poses as long as you are comfortable, or up to five minutes. After practising these exercises you should lie on your back, as shown on pages 110–111, so you can relax and do some gentle deep breathing.

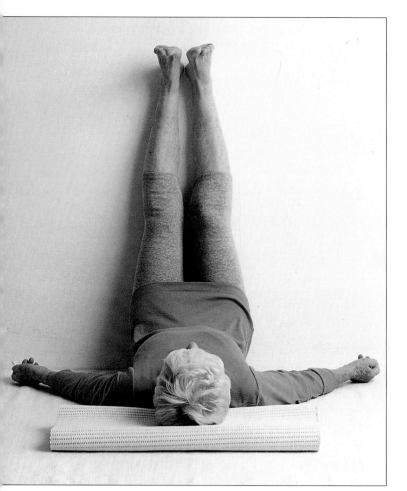

1 *Lie down at right angles to the wall. Stretch both legs up the wall and keep your knees straight. Stretch your knees as you breathe out.*

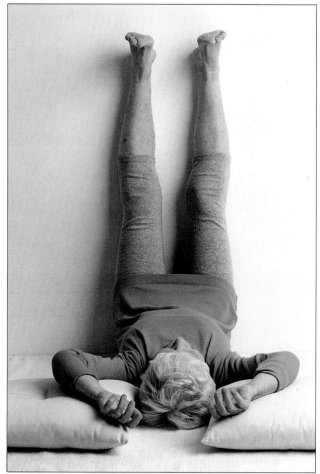

2 *Bring your arms over your head as you breathe out. Put a cushion under each arm to relax the tension in your arms and shoulders.*

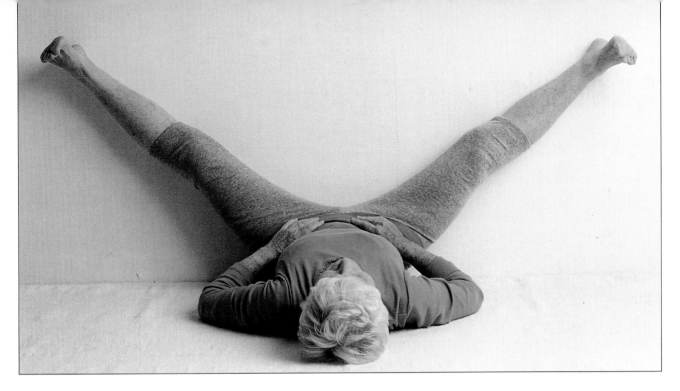

3 Spread your legs. Keep your knees straight
  and your feet equidistant from the floor.

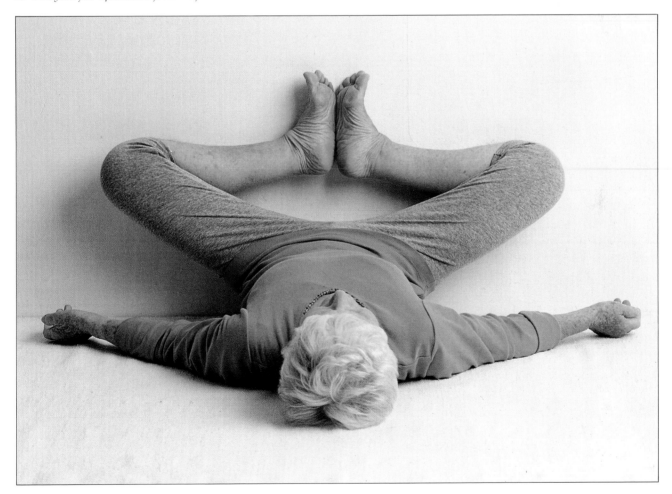

4 With your legs wide apart bend your knees
  and bring the soles of your feet together.
  Straighten your legs as in step 3.

SLEEPING POSE

YOGANIDRASANA

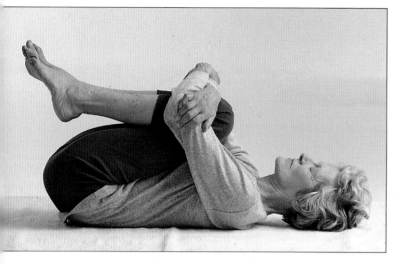

This is a relaxing, resting pose if you have long legs and a supple back. Although Sleeping Pose is done from the lying flat position, it is an advanced forward bend and is learned after you can do Tortoise (page 87). For some people it will be an easy position; for others it takes a long time to achieve, so don't try and push yourself into it too soon. Repeat the exercise with your ankles crossed over the other way and your hands clasped on the opposite side. If you have difficulty clasping your hands you can hold a belt between them. Tradition has it that this is how yogis sleep, with their feet forming a pillow and their legs wrapped around for warmth.

1 *Lie on your back on a folded blanket. Hug your knees to your chest so that your lower back stretches. Stay for a few breaths.*

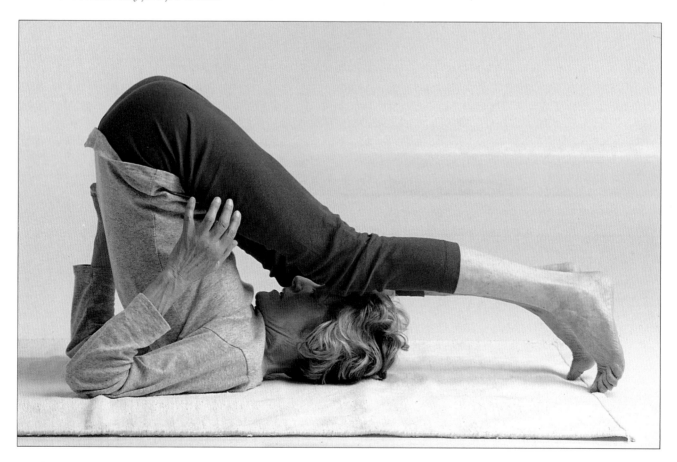

2 *As you breathe out, roll your hips up over your head, keeping your knees bent.*

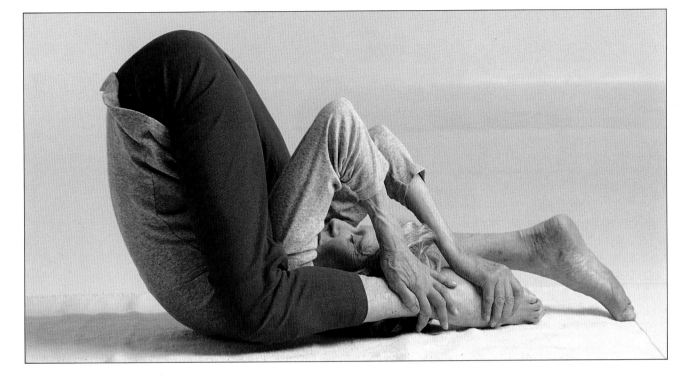

3 Bend your knees to the floor. Tuck your feet
behind your head, crossing your ankles.

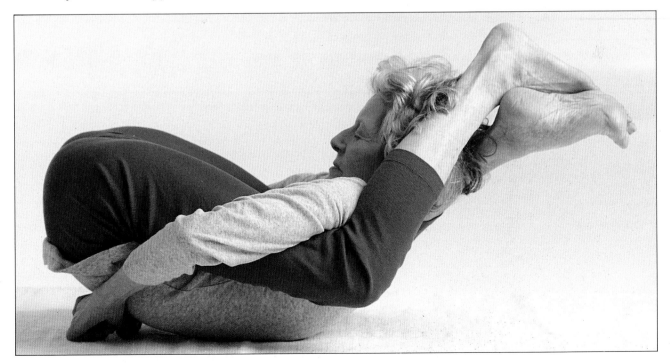

4 Reach behind your back, clasping your
hands together.

DIAMOND
VAJRASANA

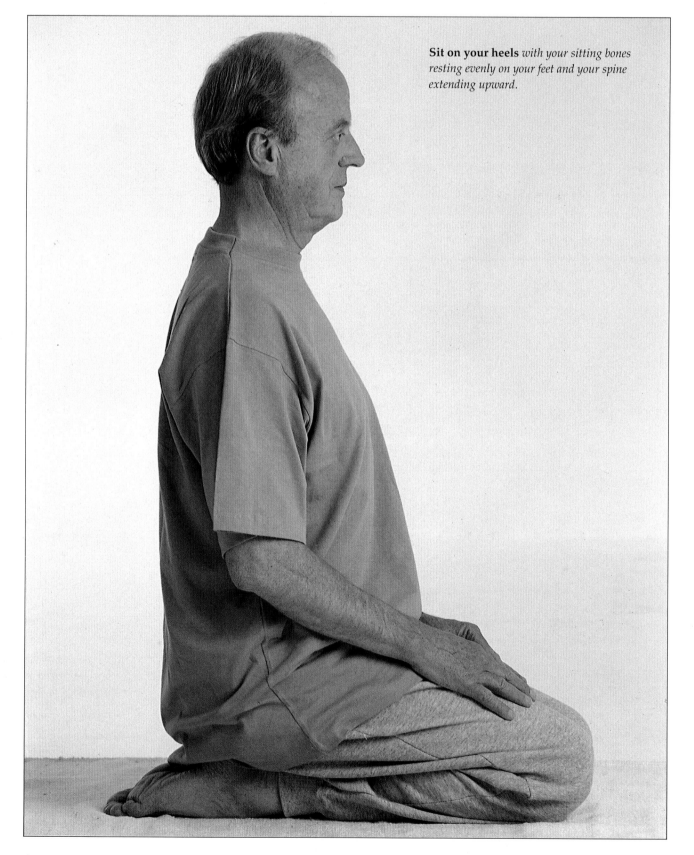

Sit on your heels *with your sitting bones resting evenly on your feet and your spine extending upward.*

This kneeling pose is one of the best positions for breathing and meditation. The pelvis is straight with the sitting bones down on your heels so that the spine can find its line of balance as you breathe. To begin with, when your hips, knees or feet may be stiff, you can try one of the variations below. You can also practice sitting with your feet tucked under.

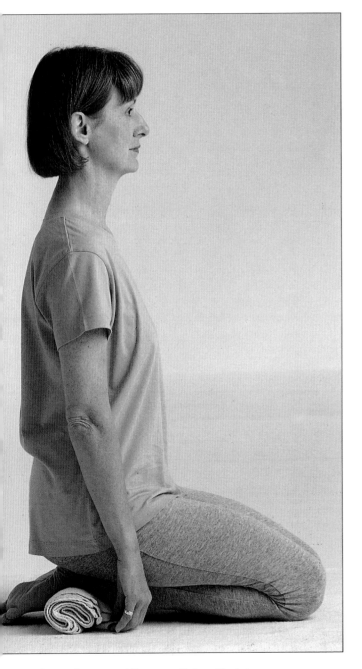

If your feet are stiff, *use a rolled-up blanket under your insteps for the first few weeks.*

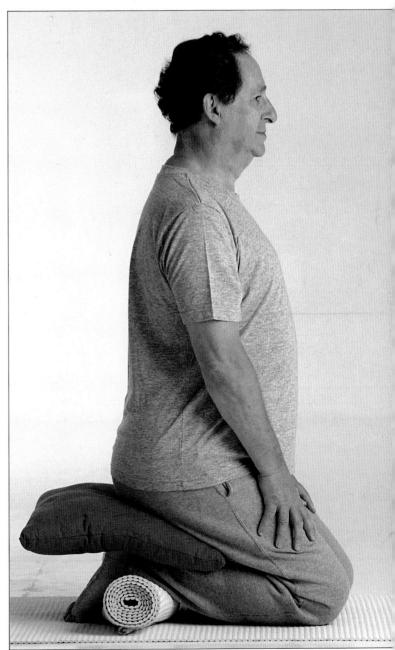

If your knees are stiff, *put a pillow between your hips and heels.*

HERO
VIRASANA

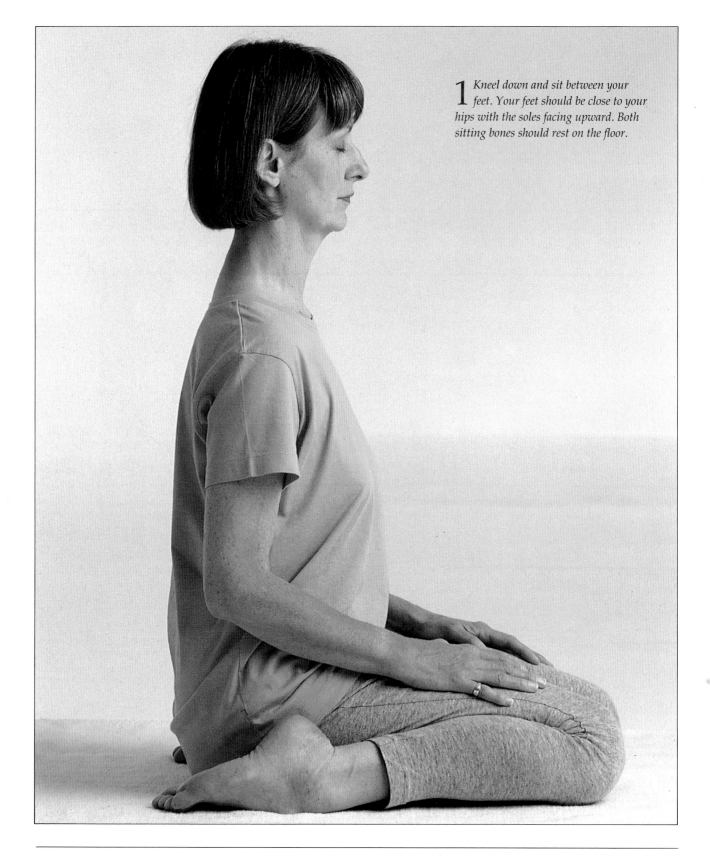

1 Kneel down and sit between your feet. Your feet should be close to your hips with the soles facing upward. Both sitting bones should rest on the floor.

In Hero you sit between your feet with your thighs turned inward. This needs flexible hips and knees so you should practice Diamond (page 62) before you attempt this. If you find it difficult at first you can put a rolled-up blanket under your feet and/or a cushion under your hips (page 63). In Hero the pelvis is pulled backward so it is not suitable for breathing and meditation unless you are very flexible.

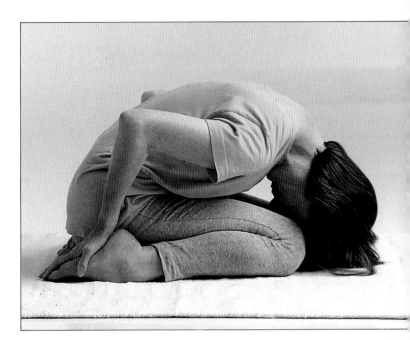

Keep your hips down *and your hands on your feet. Breathe out and bend forward.*

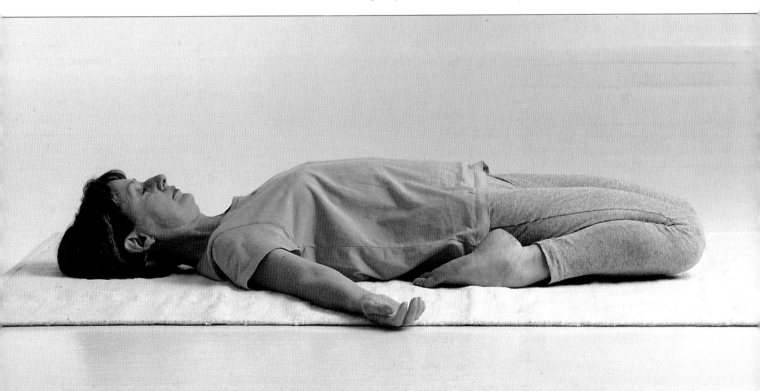

To extend back from Hero *rest back on your hands to start with, then lie flat. Tuck your* *pelvis towards your knees so that the back of your waist lengthens.*

CHILD
PINDASANA

Child pose is a relaxing, resting position and is also a preparation for Dog pose on the next page. People who find it difficult to relax lying flat on their backs in Corpse pose (page 110) find Child pose less challenging. If you have a short back or stiff hips you may not be able to go down and rest your head on the floor. In this case, put a cushion in front of you or rest your head on the seat of a low easy chair. Kneel on a mat as in Diamond (page 62) to begin the pose.

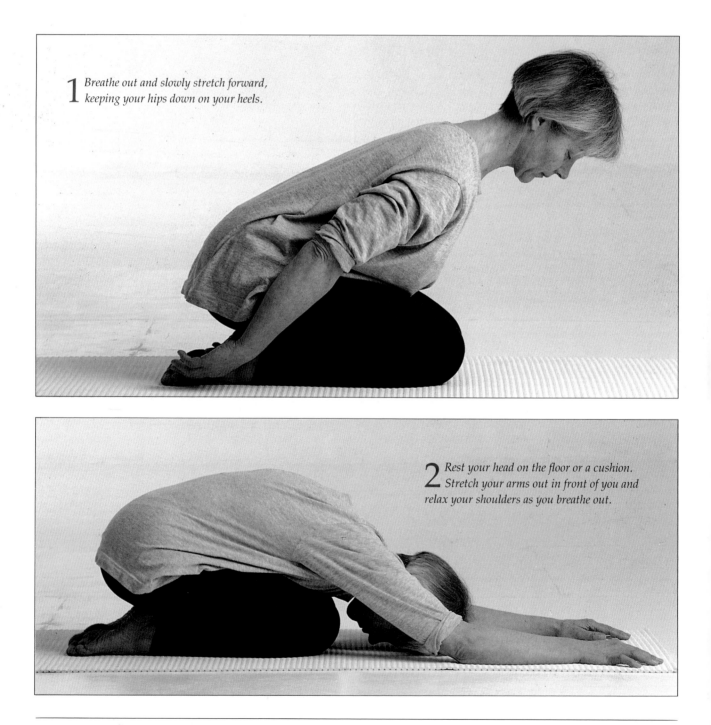

1 Breathe out and slowly stretch forward, keeping your hips down on your heels.

2 Rest your head on the floor or a cushion. Stretch your arms out in front of you and relax your shoulders as you breathe out.

DOG
SVANASANA

Dog pose is considered to be one of the most invigorating positions as it extends your spine and shoulders. It resembles a dog stretching as it gets to its feet after lying curled up. Your hands and feet are the roots in this pose and there is one long stretch from the fingers to the heels. Do not push into your shoulders and try to bring your head to the floor but let the spine lengthen and your shoulders relax as you breathe out. This is a good warm-up for the inverted poses.

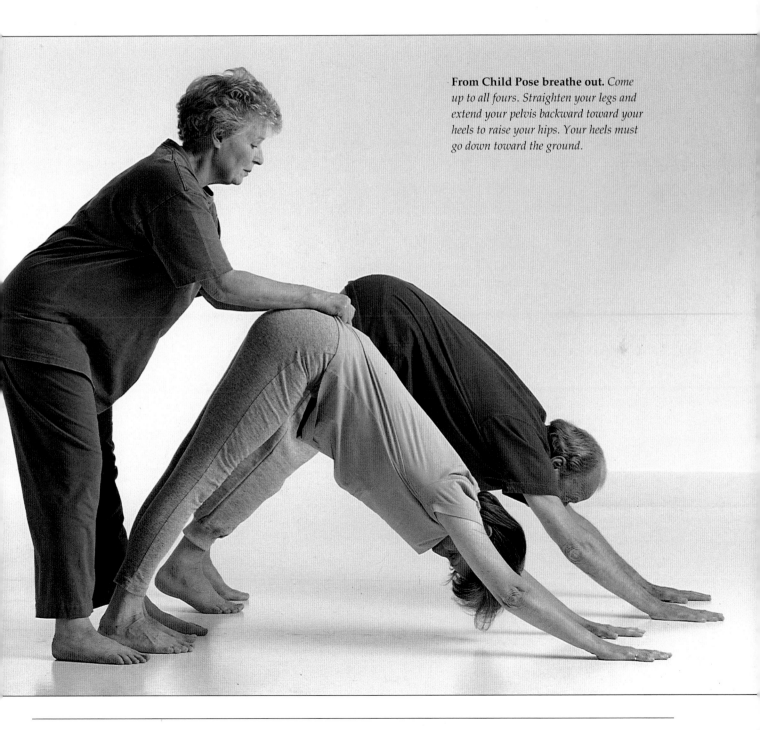

From Child Pose breathe out. *Come up to all fours. Straighten your legs and extend your pelvis backward toward your heels to raise your hips. Your heels must go down toward the ground.*

COBBLER'S POSE

BADDHA KONASANA

This sitting pose is traditionally associated with cobblers and tailors. The oldest known pose, it is depicted on the seals found in ancient sites in the Indus Valley (see page 10). The outward turn of the thighs at the hip joints, which is the key to many of the yoga poses, is where many Western people are stiff. If this is difficult, practice the stretches on page 54 (legs against the wall).

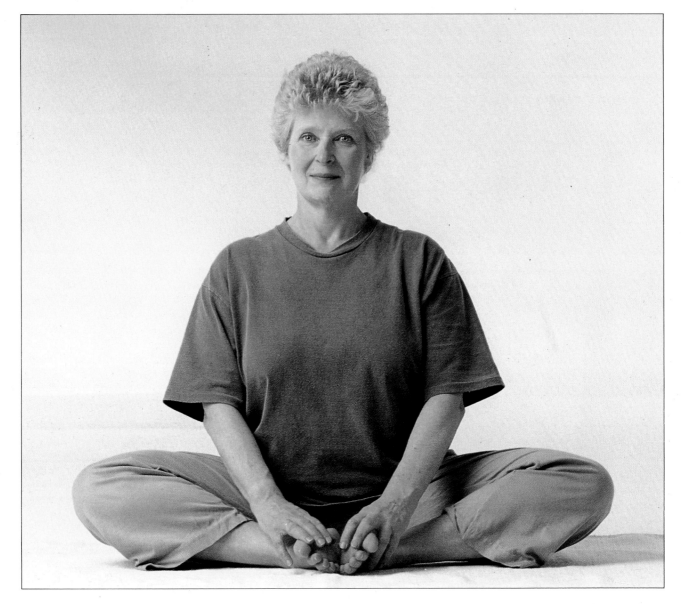

1 *Sit tall with your knees bent and feet together. Turn the soles of your feet up.*

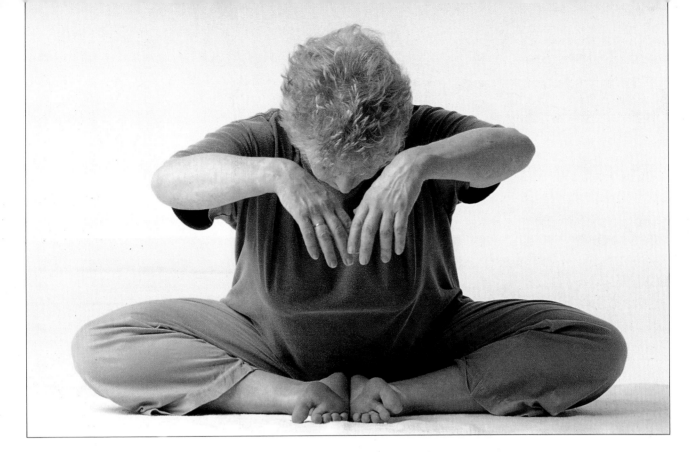

2 *Breathe out and let your thighs turn out as you stretch upward and forward.*

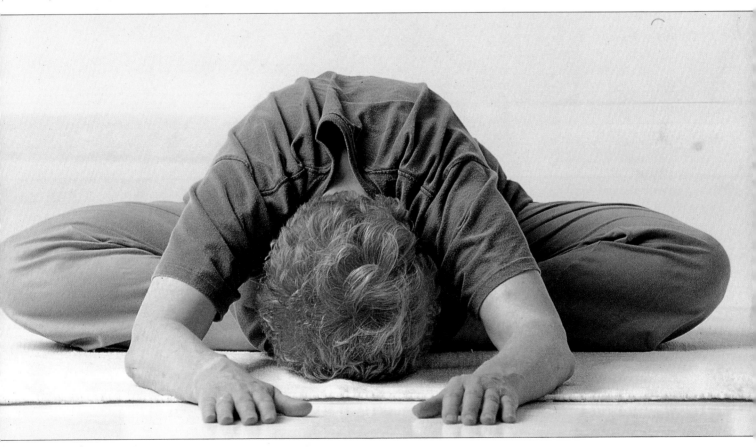

3 *Do not pull on your hands. Turning your feet out, continue to stretch forward on each exhalation until the front of your body can touch the floor.*

COW

GOMUKHASANA

This pose stretches your shoulders and also the outside of your hips. To begin with you will find it much easier to practice the arm movements when you are standing up. If it is difficult to catch your hands behind your back hold a belt between your hands. The crossed-leg position can also be practiced on its own. If your hips are stiff do not force the position. You can practice the Standing Twist (page 30) as a preparation. The crossed-arms exercise is Eagle pose.

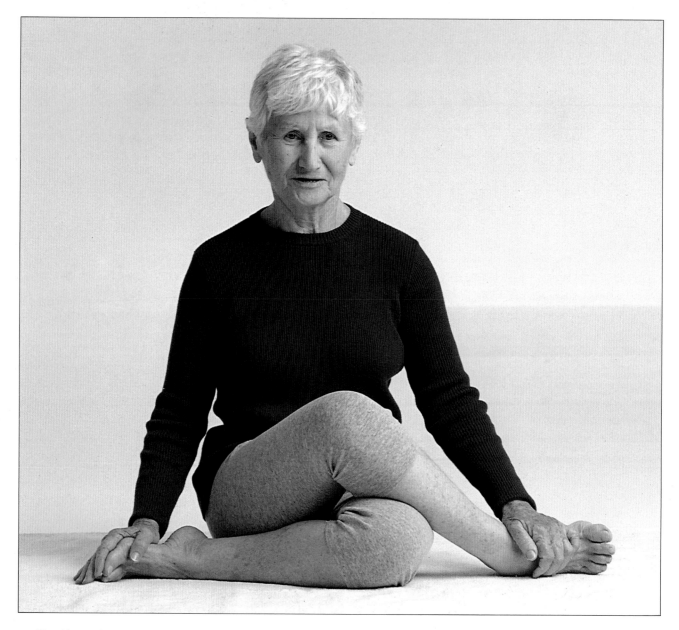

1 *Sit with your legs crossed over each other with both sitting bones touching the floor.*

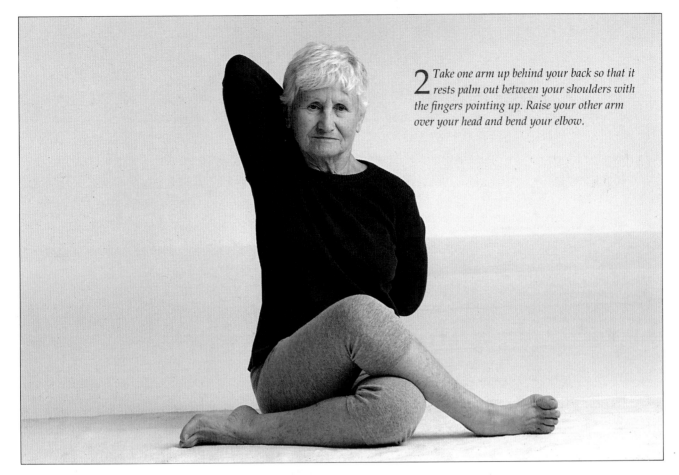

2 *Take one arm up behind your back so that it rests palm out between your shoulders with the fingers pointing up. Raise your other arm over your head and bend your elbow.*

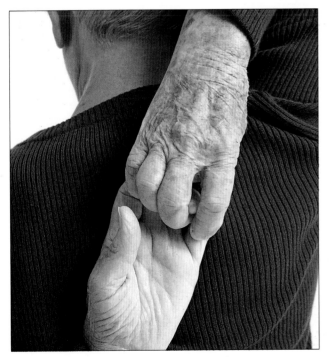

3 *Breathe out and bring your hands together. Relax your shoulders as your hands clasp.*

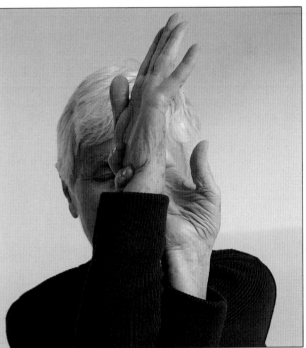

Eagle *Wrap your wrists round each other in front of you as you breathe out.*

MONKEY

HANUMANASANA

This long-legged stretch is named after the monkey general, Hanuman, who made a flying leap to fetch a healing herb which saved the life of a wounded hero in the epic poem the *Ramayana*. You need to be extraordinarily flexible to do the final stages of this beautiful pose, but

the earlier steps are excellent for loosening up stiff hips. Step 1, which stretches tight muscles round the buttock bone of the folded leg, can be helpful in some cases of lower back ache. Step 4 is an advanced pose, suitable for those with long hamstrings and flexible hips.

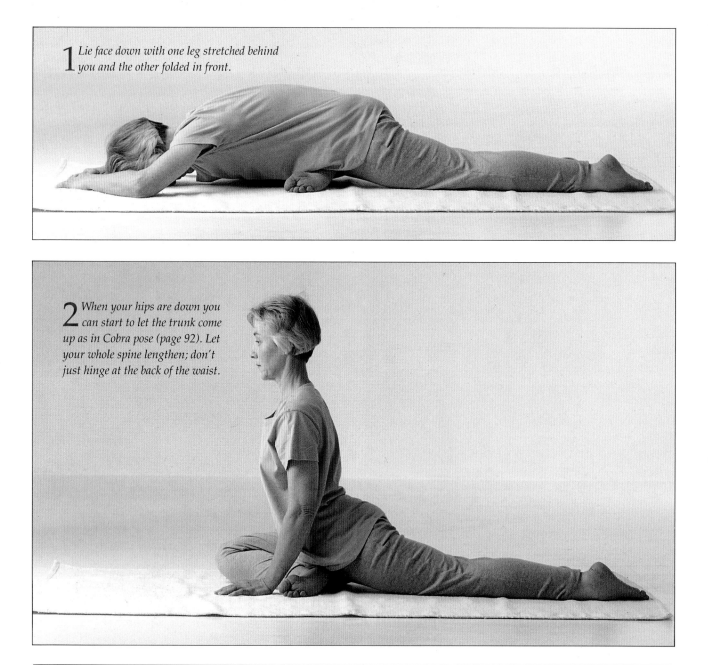

1 *Lie face down with one leg stretched behind you and the other folded in front.*

2 *When your hips are down you can start to let the trunk come up as in Cobra pose (page 92). Let your whole spine lengthen; don't just hinge at the back of the waist.*

3 *Take your front leg forward, with the knee bent, so that your thigh is parallel with your back leg. Keep your hips down and your pelvis straight.*

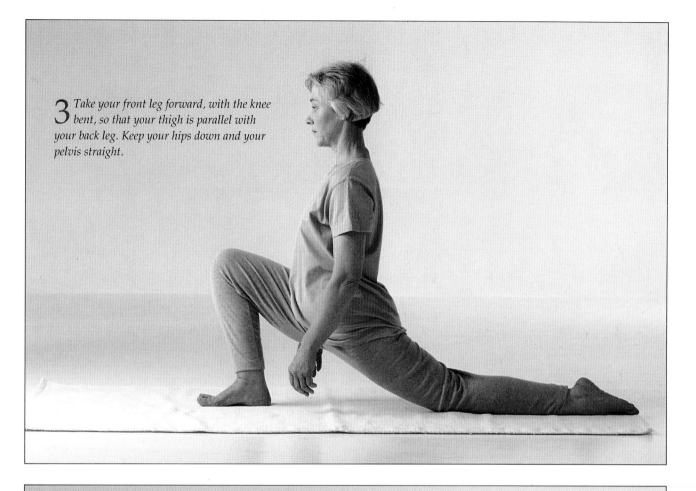

4 *Keep your hips down and let your front leg straighten. Your back leg must be turned in so that your knee faces the floor and your hips remain straight.*

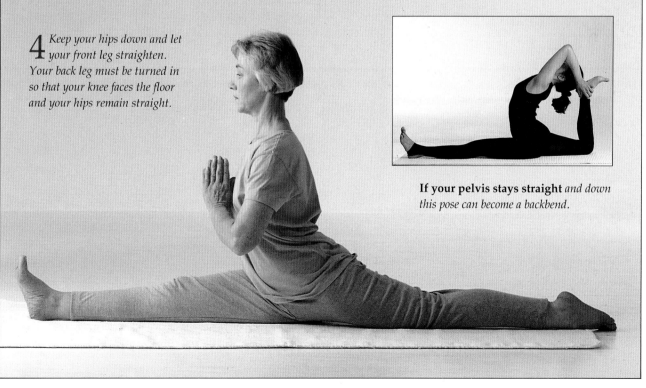

If your pelvis stays straight *and down this pose can become a backbend.*

LOTUS
PADMASANA

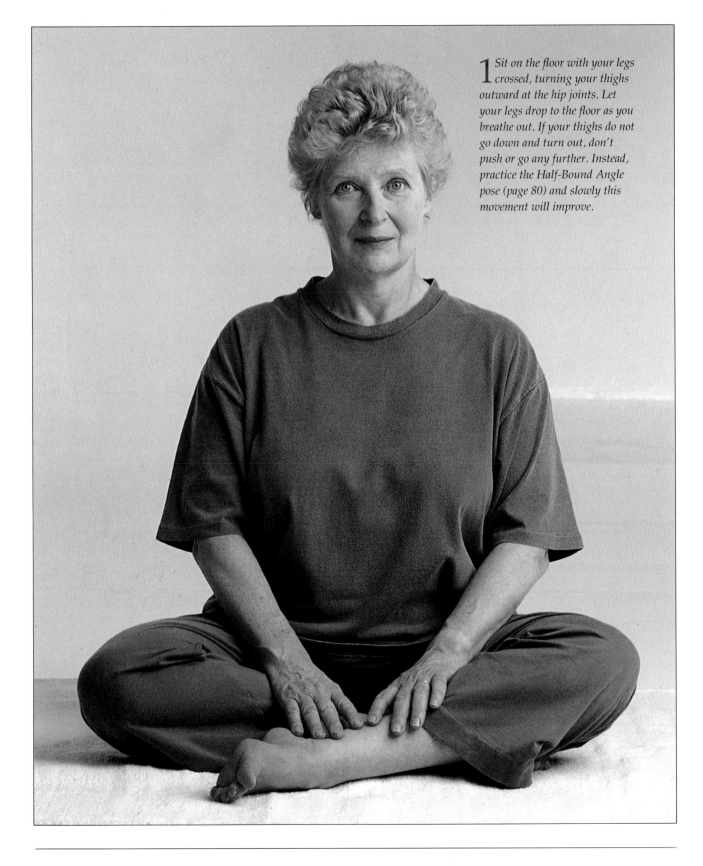

1 *Sit on the floor with your legs crossed, turning your thighs outward at the hip joints. Let your legs drop to the floor as you breathe out. If your thighs do not go down and turn out, don't push or go any further. Instead, practice the Half-Bound Angle pose (page 80) and slowly this movement will improve.*

The lotus symbolizes spiritual search and enlightenment. In this pose, the pelvis is held straight by the position of the feet which are folded on to the thighs, so that the spine can balance in its four curves. For many people who have spent a lifetime sitting on chairs this is not an easy pose at first, but once it is mastered it is the best way to sit for any length of time. The base of this *asana* is completely stable, allowing the upper body to sit both straight and relaxed. In this pose the rotation comes from the hip joints and not the knees. Cross your legs the other way every time you practice, to avoid developing an imbalance in your hip joints.

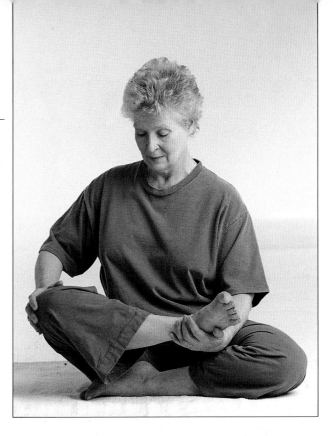

2 *Turning at the hip, lift one leg and bring the foot up to rest on the opposite thigh. This is Half-Lotus,* ardha padmasana.

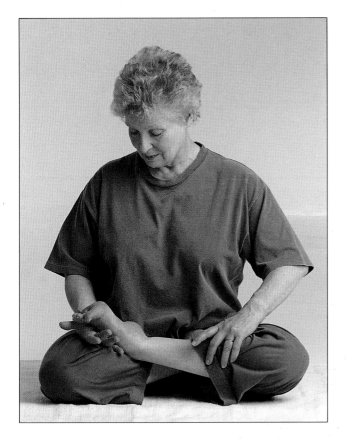

3 *Breathe out, let your hips drop as you sit up, lift the other leg and bring the foot on top of the opposite thigh. Keep the knee down.*

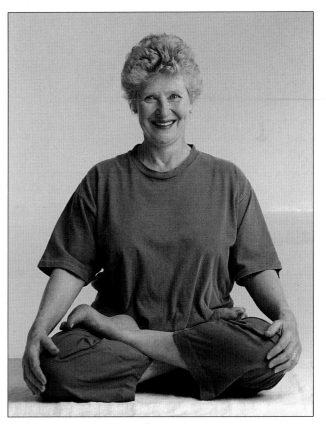

4 *Sit tall with your back straight, let your shoulders relax and keep your hands resting on your knees.*

MORE LOTUS POSES
PADMASANA

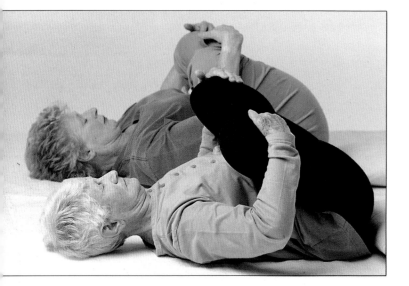

From Lotus you can bend backward, forward and twist. All these movements stretch the spine away from the pelvis as you breathe out, helping you sit tall with your hips down and your body in line with gravity. In the Fish pose below (*matsyasana*), put a cushion under your thighs to begin with. This is to ensure that your lower spine lengthens as your legs go down toward the floor. The back of your waist should only curve up a little in this position. Remember to practice these poses with your legs crossed on a different side each time. These exercises are good warm-ups for breathing or meditation in Lotus.

Lie down with *your legs in Lotus. Breathe out and bring your knees toward your chest, letting the back of your waist lengthen.*

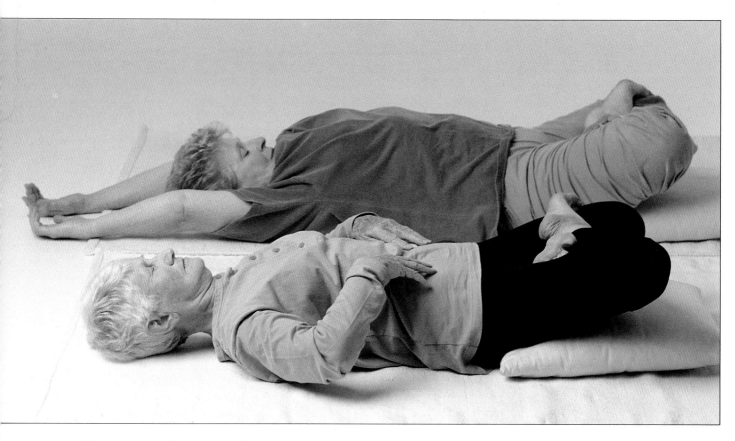

Fish (*matsyasana*) *Breathe out and bring your knees down toward the floor.*

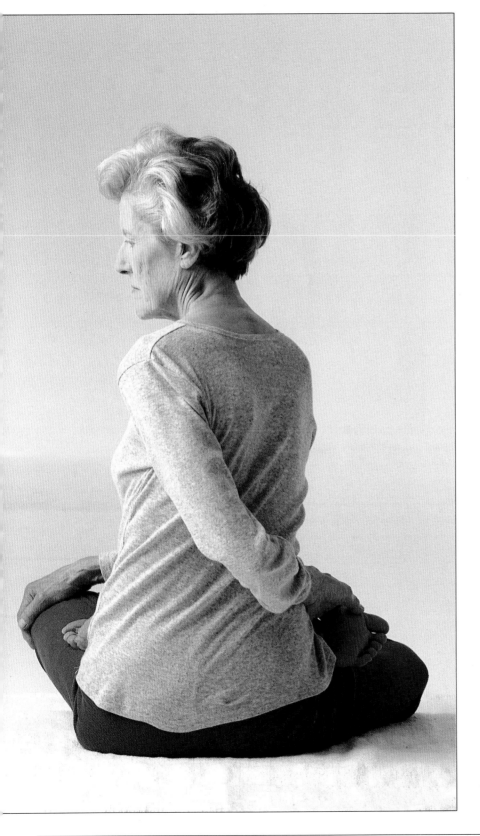

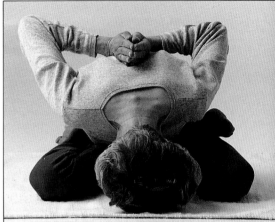

Sit in Lotus *and take your hands behind your back (page 28). Breathe out then bend forward, keeping your hips down so that your spine lengthens.*

Sit in Lotus, *breathe out, turn toward the hip of the upper leg and take your arm behind you to hold the top of the foot which is uppermost.*

SITTING STRETCH

PASCHIMOTTANASANA

This is the classic forward bend. Make sure that you have your weight evenly distributed on your sitting bones before you begin and that your legs are stretching equally away from you. As in the Standing Forward Bend (page 20) your back should not collapse and shorten but must lengthen as you go forward. Do not strain to touch your feet or pull on your arms but let your hips stay well down and lengthen upward as you breathe out. At first you may have to tighten your thigh muscles to straighten your knees but eventually you will be able to go forward easily without straining. If you cannot reach your toes, loop a belt around your feet and hold that instead. Keep the back of your neck long as you stretch up. If you are stiff, you are advised to practice the Standing Forward Bend before you do this pose.

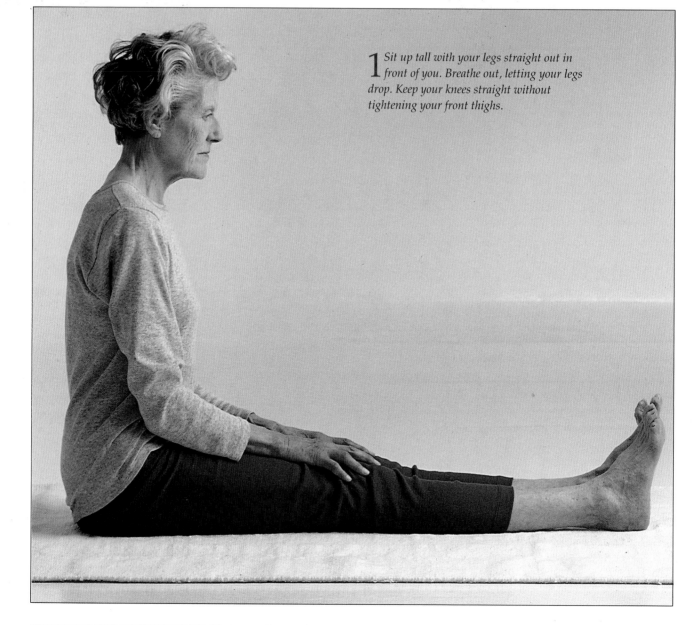

1 *Sit up tall with your legs straight out in front of you. Breathe out, letting your legs drop. Keep your knees straight without tightening your front thighs.*

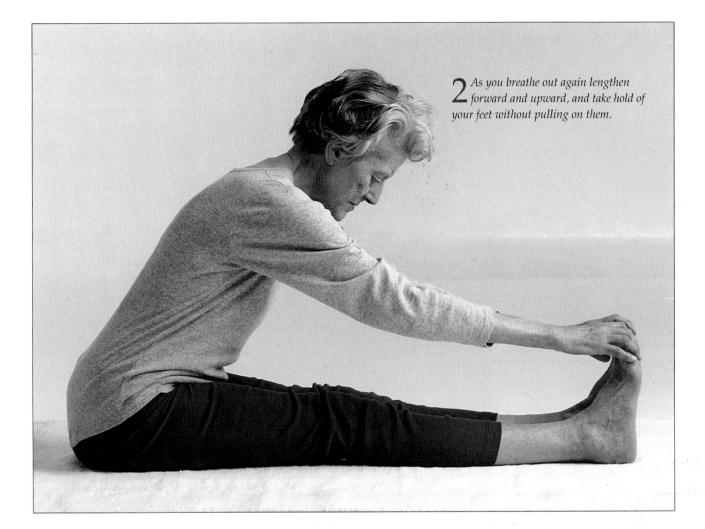

2 *As you breathe out again lengthen forward and upward, and take hold of your feet without pulling on them.*

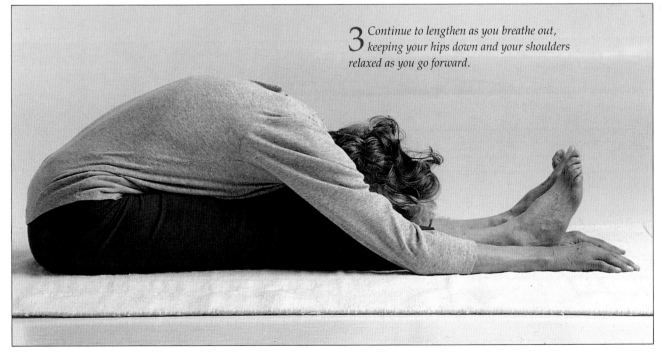

3 *Continue to lengthen as you breathe out, keeping your hips down and your shoulders relaxed as you go forward.*

HALF-BOUND ANGLE
JANU SIRSASANA

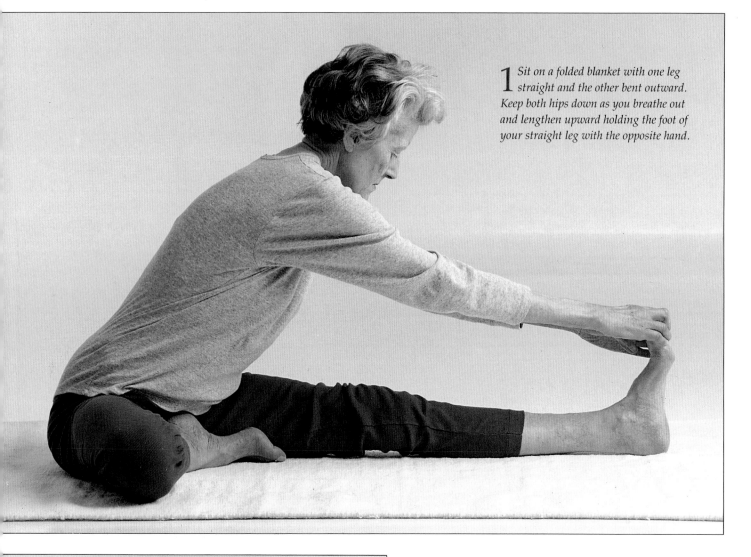

1 Sit on a folded blanket with one leg straight and the other bent outward. Keep both hips down as you breathe out and lengthen upward holding the foot of your straight leg with the opposite hand.

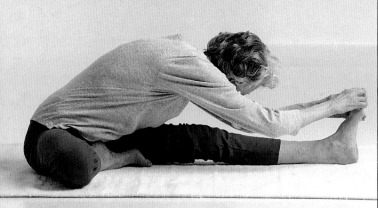

2 Breathe out, bend forward, keep your hips down and your arms and shoulders passive.

In this sitting forward stretch your sitting bones and your bent leg have to stay down as you lengthen forward. This needs a good outward rotation at the hip joint. Until your bent leg can touch the floor stay in step 1, lengthening upward and dropping your thigh down as you breathe out. Try putting a cushion under your thigh to help it relax. Hold a belt looped around your foot if you can't reach it with your hand.

HALF-HERO
TRIANGMUKHAIKAPADA PASCHIMOTTANASANA

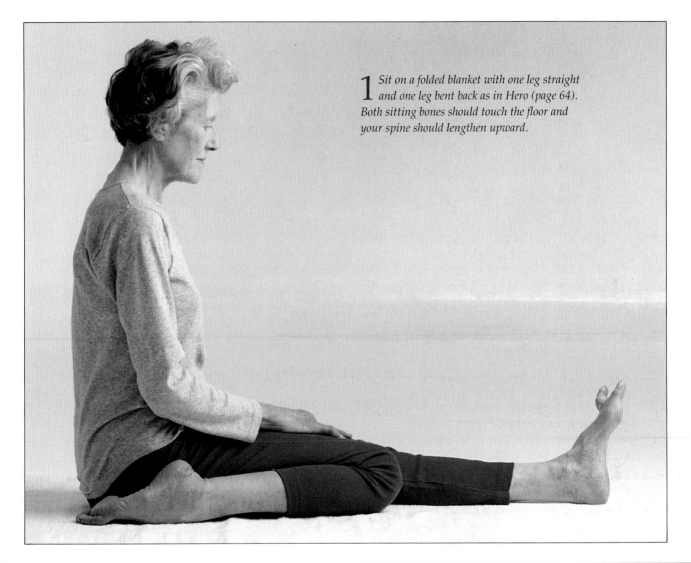

1 *Sit on a folded blanket with one leg straight and one leg bent back as in Hero (page 64). Both sitting bones should touch the floor and your spine should lengthen upward.*

In this pose most people find it difficult to keep their weight on both sitting bones as the hip of the folded leg tends to come up. So spend time in step 1, letting your pelvis drop as you breathe out and stretch upward. The foot of the folded leg should be close to your hip with the toes pointing backward. If your feet are stiff, practice Diamond with a blanket under them (page 62). Repeat the pose on the other side.

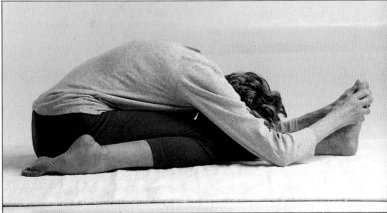

2 *Breathe out and stretch upward and forward to hold the foot of the straight leg.*

FORWARD ANGLE POSE

UPAVISTHA KONASANA

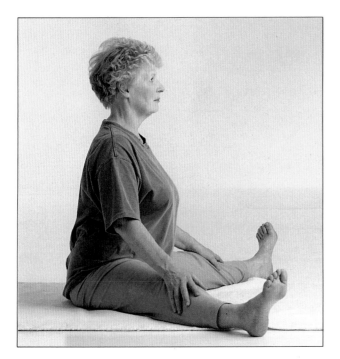

You can use step 1 of this sitting forward bend for breathing or meditation if you have injured knees. It is, however, a difficult pose if the muscles at the back of your legs are tight as this pulls the pelvis back, preventing you from sitting up straight. In this case, sit with your back against a wall. Don't try to go forward until you can sit straight and unsupported.

1 *Sit with your legs wide apart, your knees and back straight.*

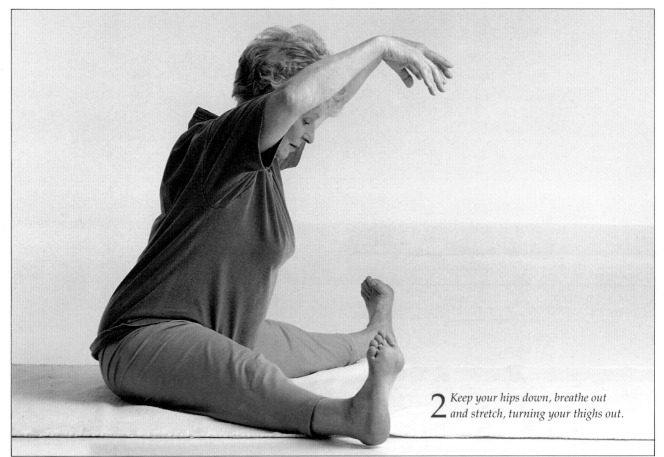

2 *Keep your hips down, breathe out and stretch, turning your thighs out.*

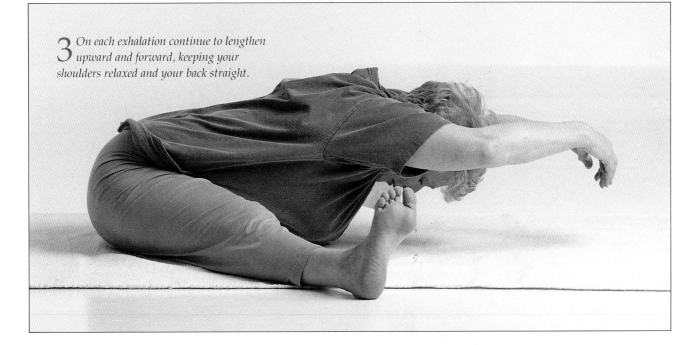

3 On each exhalation continue to lengthen upward and forward, keeping your shoulders relaxed and your back straight.

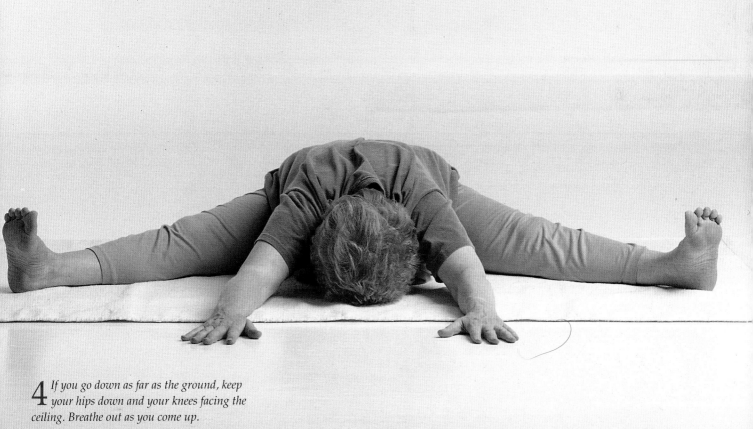

4 If you go down as far as the ground, keep your hips down and your knees facing the ceiling. Breathe out as you come up.

HERON
KROUNCHASANA

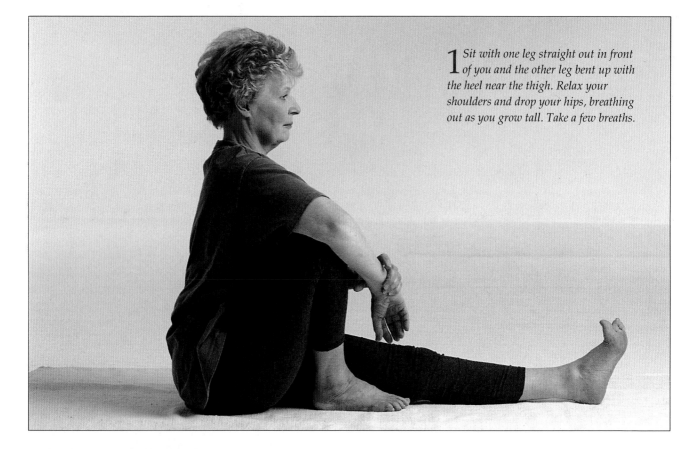

1 *Sit with one leg straight out in front of you and the other leg bent up with the heel near the thigh. Relax your shoulders and drop your hips, breathing out as you grow tall. Take a few breaths.*

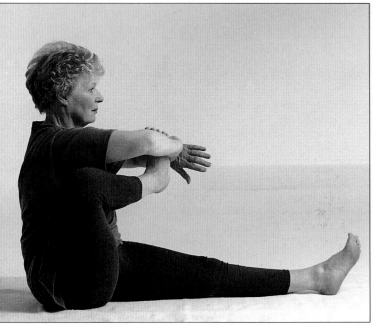

2 *Breathe out. Raise the bent leg by holding your foot and drawing it toward you.*

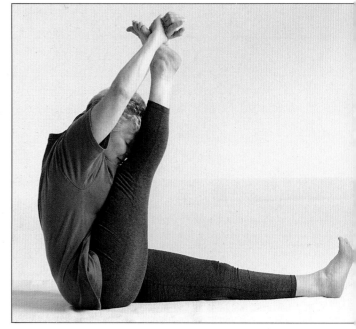

3 *Bring your foot higher as you breathe out. Keep your trunk in contact with your leg.*

First of all, learn this pose with one leg raised, as shown on the left-hand page. When you can do this easily, try taking both legs up at the same time, as shown below. When doing this sit with your back near a support, as you may tend to fall backward to start with. The movement in this *asana* is from the base of your spine. Keep your hips down, your arms bent and let the pose grow slowly as you breathe out, keeping your shoulders relaxed. Go slowly and do not progress beyond step 2 at first.

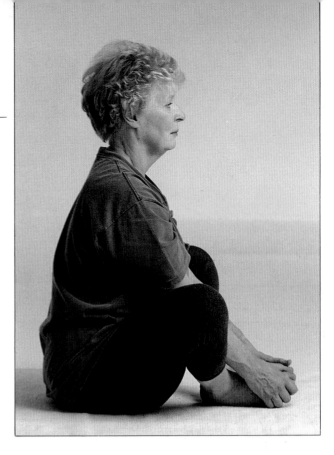

1 *Sit with your knees bent, holding your feet close to you. Keep your back straight.*

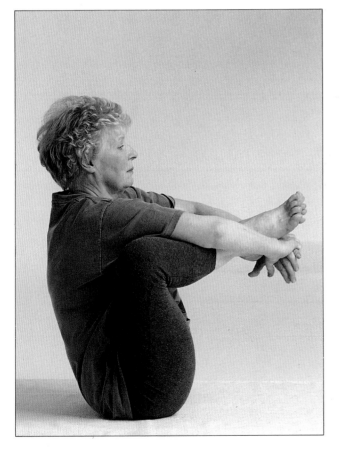

2 *Breathe out and lift your feet toward you. Your knees come toward your armpits.*

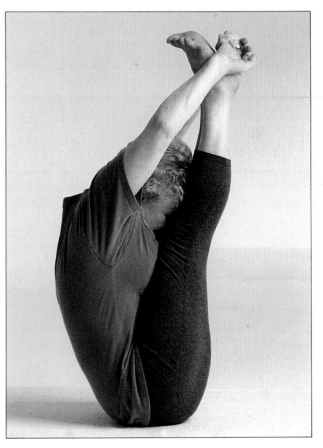

3 *With each exhalation raise your feet higher. Keep your thighs close to your trunk.*

TORTOISE

KURMASANA

Tortoise is a difficult forward bend that requires a supple spine, shoulders and hips, particularly for the final step – the Sleeping Tortoise (*supta kurmasana*). Practice the other forward bends before you try this so you understand how to keep your hips down and lengthen your spine as you breathe out. If you wait for your upper back to lengthen and your chest to drop you will be able to move your arms easily. Practice step 4 with your ankles crossed each way.

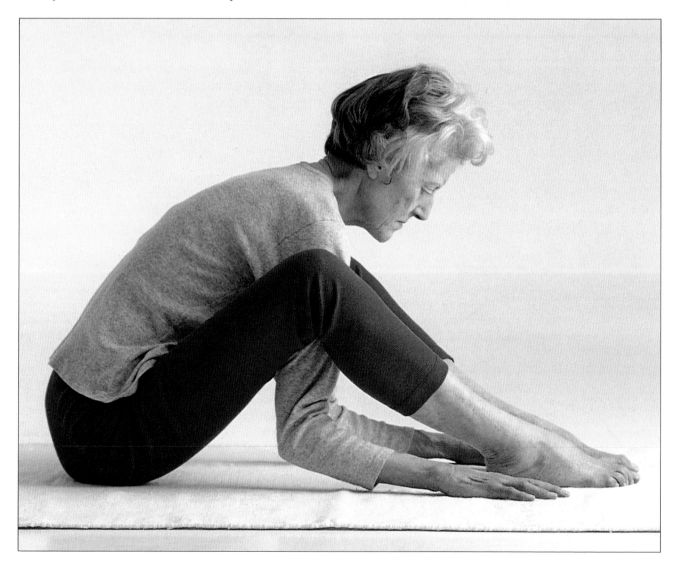

1 *Sit with your knees bent and your feet hip-width apart. Keep your hips down and* stretch up as you breathe out and go forward. Drop your elbows down between your knees.

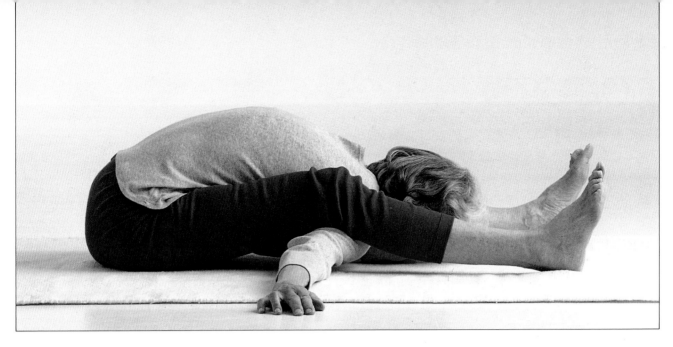

2 *Continue to lengthen forward as you breathe out. When your knees are above* your shoulders turn your arms so they reach under your knees with the palms facing down.

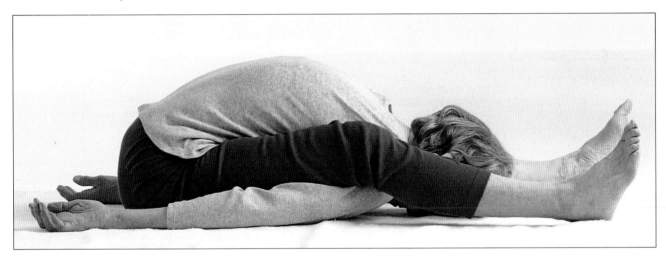

3 *Keeping your knees close to your trunk, breathe out again and, turning your arms* so that the palms face upward, take your hands back by your hips.

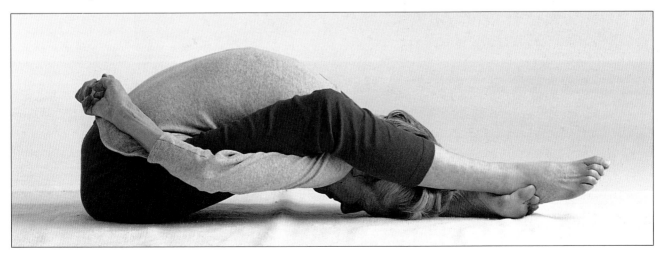

4 *Bend your elbows and catch your hands behind your back. Raising your head, draw* your feet toward you and cross your ankles. Drop your head between your shins.

LOCUST

SALABHASANA

This pose is not as simple as it seems. If you compress the back of the waist and neck it is easy to bend backward, but in backbending movements the whole of the spine should lengthen and bend. For this you need strong back thigh muscles to hold the pelvis down, so that the spine can lengthen toward the head as the upper back straightens. The movement has to come from the spine as you breathe, so when you breathe out to come up into the pose, pull your abdomen and solar plexus inward and relax your shoulders.

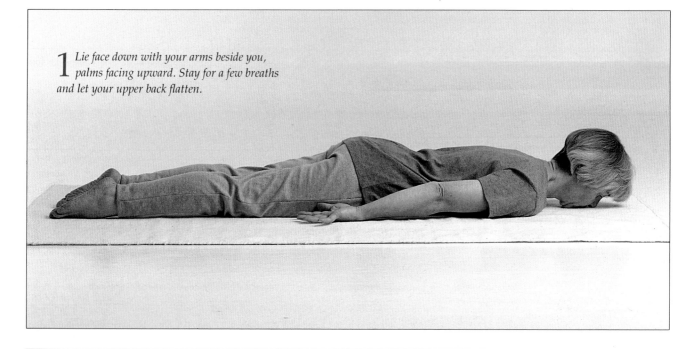

1 Lie face down with your arms beside you, palms facing upward. Stay for a few breaths and let your upper back flatten.

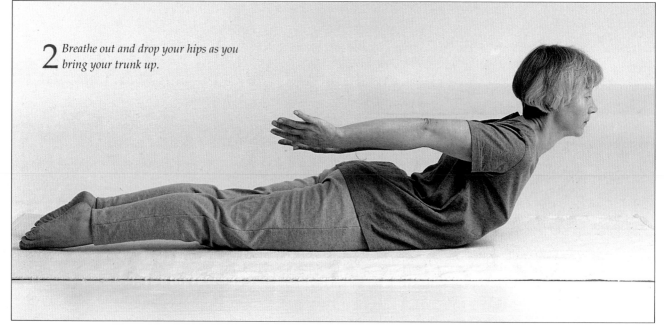

2 Breathe out and drop your hips as you bring your trunk up.

BOW
DHANURASANA

In this pose the bowstring pulls on each end of the bow, which bends evenly. Your arms and legs stretch away from the trunk and the spine lengthens as it bends as a whole; it should not just hinge at the back of the waist. This action is similar to the Wheel pose (sometimes called Reversed Bow) where your hands and feet go down into the earth to complete a circle under the ground (page 91). As in the Locust, draw your abdomen inward so the movement comes from your spine. Go into the pose as you breathe out and keep your chin in to lengthen your neck.

1 *Lie on the floor face downward. Breathe out and, dropping your hips, bend your knees and catch your ankles. Keep your chin in.*

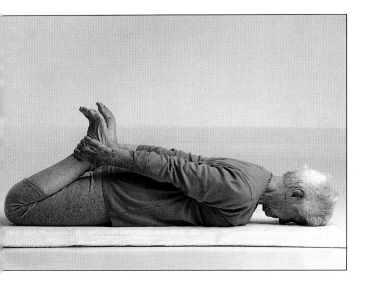

2 *Breathe out and lift up. The movement comes from the spine and not from the shoulders. Keep your neck and face relaxed.*

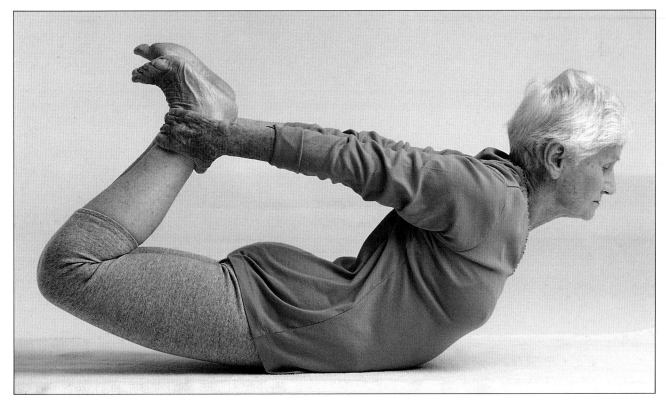

BRIDGE
SETU BANDHA SARVANGASANA

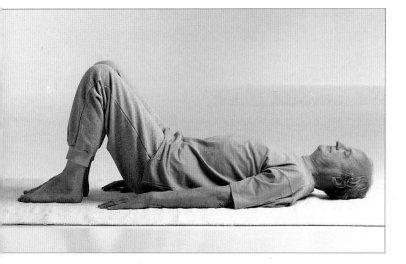

This backbend should resemble the span of a bridge; your spine should lengthen in one long smooth curve and not just bend in the middle. As you breathe out to come up into the pose, drop the back of your waist down and scoop your hips up so that the crease under the buttocks tightens as they lift. Your heels must stay down as you come up into the arch. These give the bridge the strong supports it needs for you to be able to stretch easily. As you do this, keep your shoulders relaxed.

1 *Lie flat with your knees bent up. Your feet should be hip-width apart and parallel.*

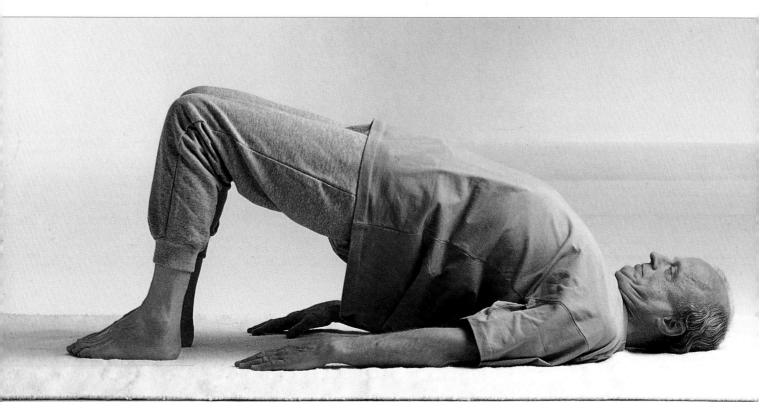

2 *Keeping your feet flat on the floor, breathe out and lift your hips up to form an arch in your spine. Come down gently and hug your knees to your chest (page 55).*

WHEEL

URDHVA DHANURASANA

When your spine extends freely in the Wheel position it brings a marvelous feeling of energy. It is a particularly rejuvenating and invigorating pose. For this your spine, shoulders, and hips have to be strong and flexible so it is not a pose to be attempted by beginners. If you try it before you are ready, it merely compresses the spinal curves and makes you feel exhausted. Spend some time in step 1 before you push up on your hands and feet. These are the roots of the pose; as you come up keep them down firmly so that the curve of the waist lengthens as you lift up.

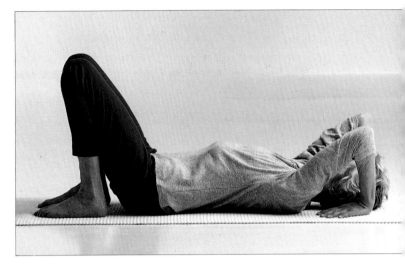

1 *Lie with your back flat, feet hip-width apart and your hands under your shoulders.*

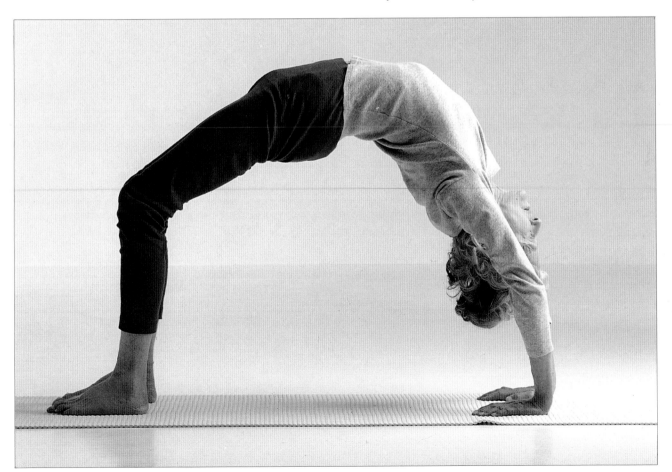

2 *Breathe out and drop your waist as you lift your hips. Keeping your heels and wrists down, come up into the pose. Hold for a few breaths then come down and hug your knees.*

COBRA

B H U J A N G A S A N A

Cobra looks simple but it is not an easy pose to
get right. There is a temptation in this pose to
push yourself up on your hands and compress
the curve at the back of the waist. Therefore,
learn the action in the Locust pose (page 88) so
that you can feel the backbending movement
coming from the spine as you breathe out and
lengthen your upper back. The Cobra is a snake:
keep this image in your mind as you do the pose.

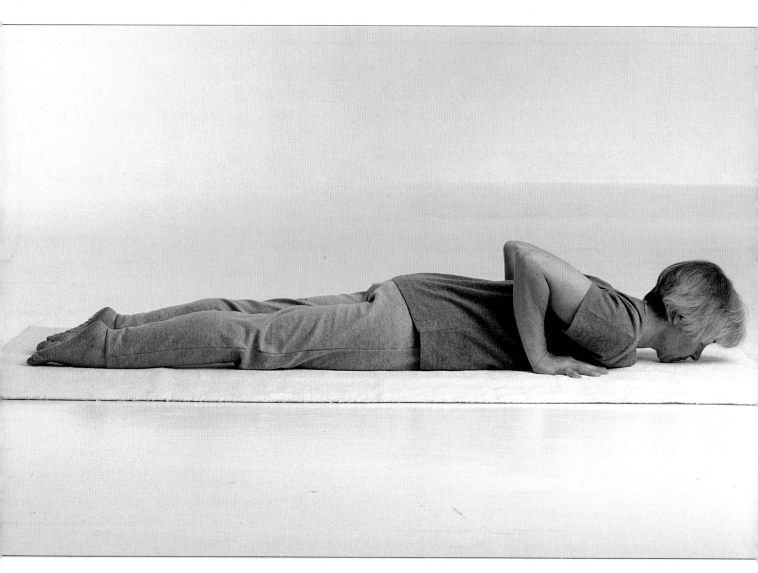

1 *Lie face down, hands under your shoulders
with the fingers facing forward.*

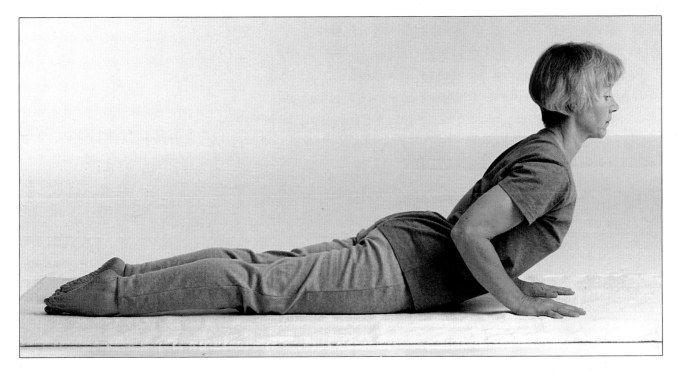

2 *As you breathe out drop your hips and lengthen forward as you come up.*

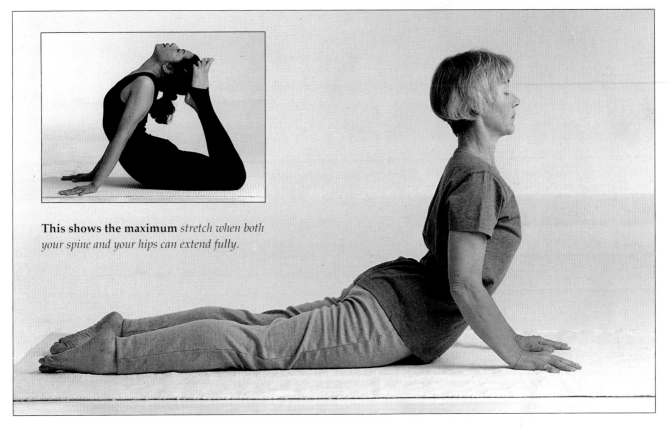

This shows the maximum *stretch when both your spine and your hips can extend fully.*

3 *Lengthen as you breathe out, keeping your buttock muscles strong.*

SAGE

MARICHYASANA

This pose is, in Sanskrit, named after the wise man Marichi. It can be done either as a forward bend, taking your head down toward your straight knee, or as the twisting movement shown here. You need good flexibility in your hips for this position, both with legs bent and straight, so it is not a pose that is suitable for beginners. As you sit with one leg straight on the ground, the arm on the opposite side is

twined round the knee which is bent up toward the chest. In this position the spine can turn as you stretch up to sit straight. The position of your arm helps your upper back to straighten and it is an excellent pose if you have a tendency to stoop. The turn has to come from the spine as you breathe out, so resist the temptation to push against your knee with your elbow. Go slowly; it may take time to clasp your hands together.

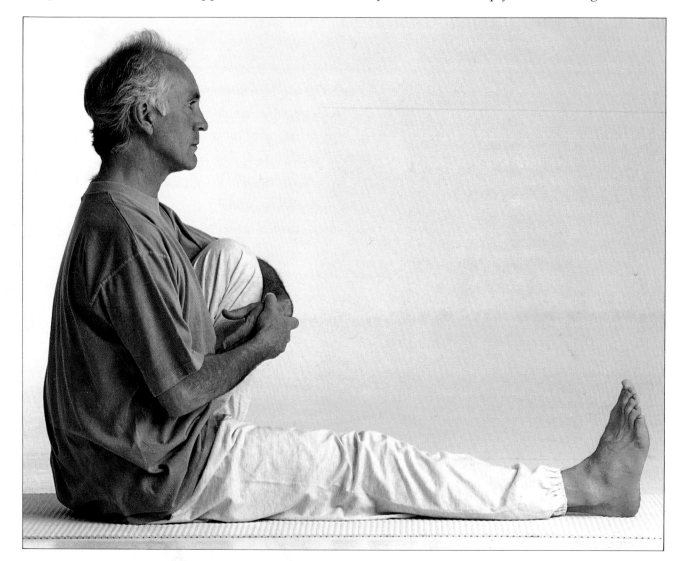

1 *Sit on the floor with your right leg straight out in front of you and your left leg bent up so that the heel is close to the back of the thigh.*

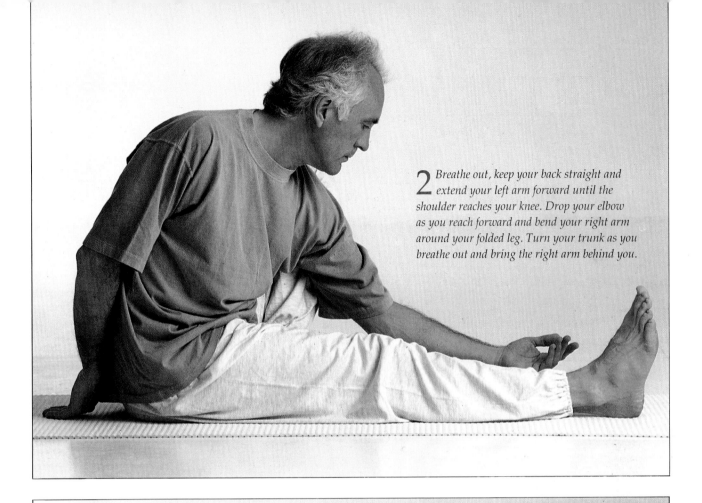

2 Breathe out, keep your back straight and extend your left arm forward until the shoulder reaches your knee. Drop your elbow as you reach forward and bend your right arm around your folded leg. Turn your trunk as you breathe out and bring the right arm behind you.

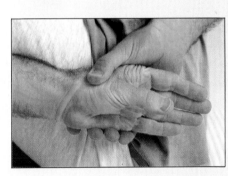

3 Clasp your hands behind your back, lengthen your spine, sit up straight and turn. Keep your hands relaxed and hold the wrist of the other hand. If you find this difficult, hold a belt between your hands to start with. Repeat on the other side.

SAGE TWIST

MARICHYASANA

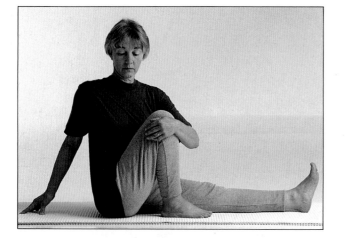

Sage Twist has a more intense movement than Sage pose (page 94). As in the other twists you have to lengthen, growing tall as you turn.
In Sage Twist your bent knee should come into your armpit as you do this. If you have a long back and short legs this may make this pose difficult, in which case do Lotus Twist (page 76) or Wide Angle Twist (page 100) instead.

1 *Sit with one leg straight and the other bent up with the foot close to the back thigh.*

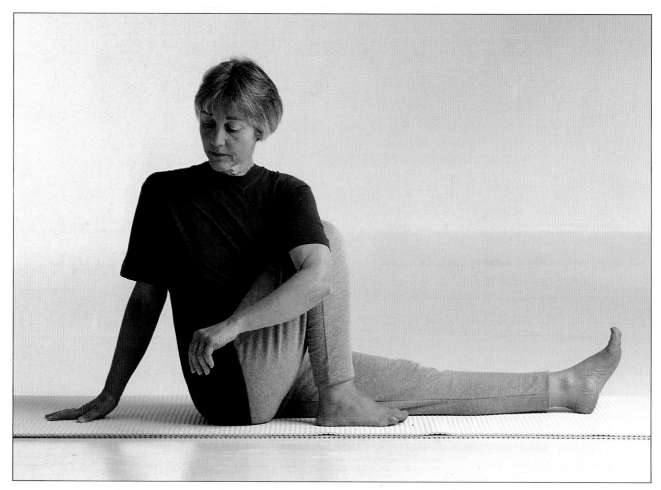

2 *Breathe out. Turn toward your bent leg, letting the arm drop outside your thigh.*

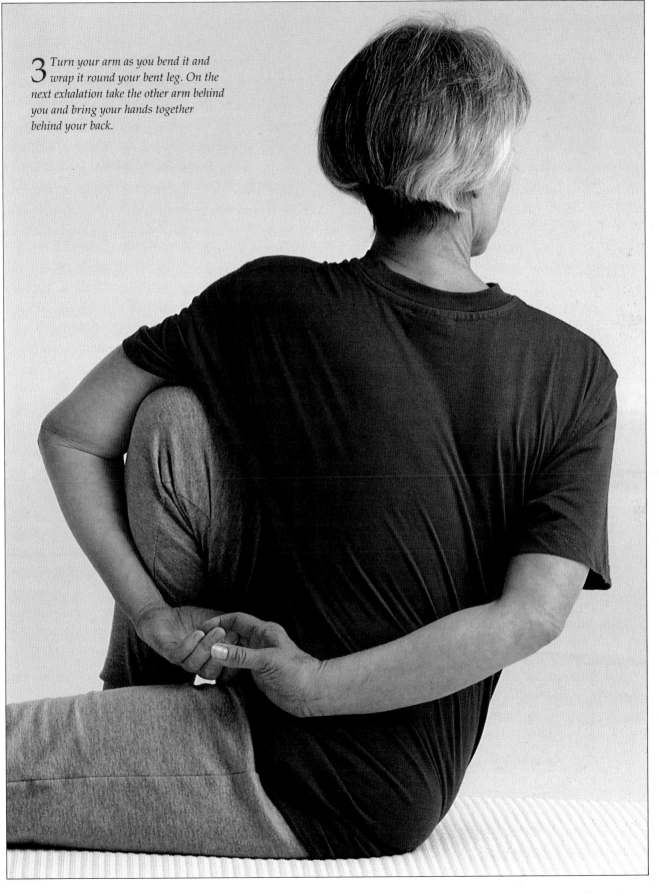

3 *Turn your arm as you bend it and wrap it round your bent leg. On the next exhalation take the other arm behind you and bring your hands together behind your back.*

HALF-SAGE TWIST

ARDHA MATSYENDRASANA

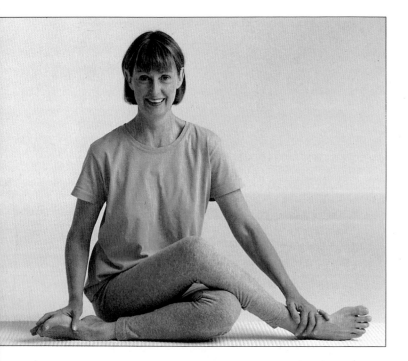

This is a difficult twist and you should be able to do Cow (page 70) and Sage Twist (page 96) before you try it. In this twist your body folds inward and then releases and opens out as the spine turns and lengthens. The center of the pose is strong and compact. There is a legend that Matsyendra was a fish who learned the secret of yoga by overhearing the god Siva teaching his consort, and was transformed into a man.

1 *Sit with the legs folded as in Cow (page 70). Keep your hips down and shoulders relaxed.*

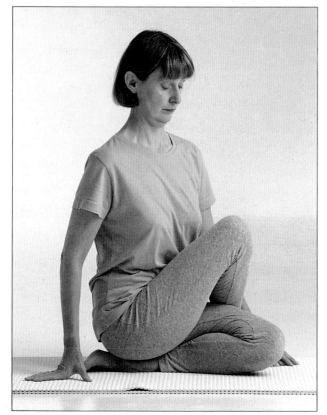

2 *Lift your hips and sit on the inner curve of your left foot, bringing in your right knee.*

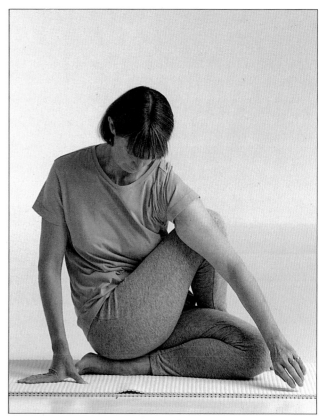

3 *Turn right and drop your left arm outside your right leg, turning back your palm.*

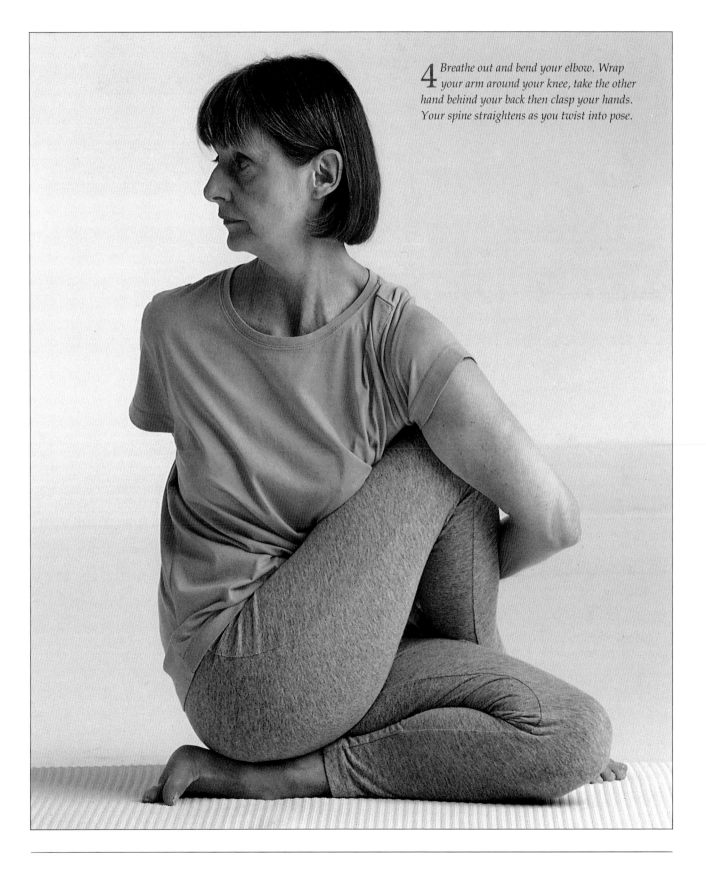

4 *Breathe out and bend your elbow. Wrap your arm around your knee, take the other hand behind your back then clasp your hands. Your spine straightens as you twist into pose.*

WIDE ANGLE TWIST

PARIVRTTA UPAVISTHA KONASANA

You need to be able to bend into the Forward Angle Pose (page 82) before you try this twist. All the twisting movements come from your spine and you have to be careful not to push with your elbow to lever yourself into the position as this tightens your shoulders and blocks the movement of the upper back. Keep your hips down as you go into the pose and turn your legs outward at the hips so that your knees continue to face the ceiling throughout. This pose is particularly good if you are stiff on one side of the trunk or hip. In this case, stay in the pose longer to extend the stiff side.

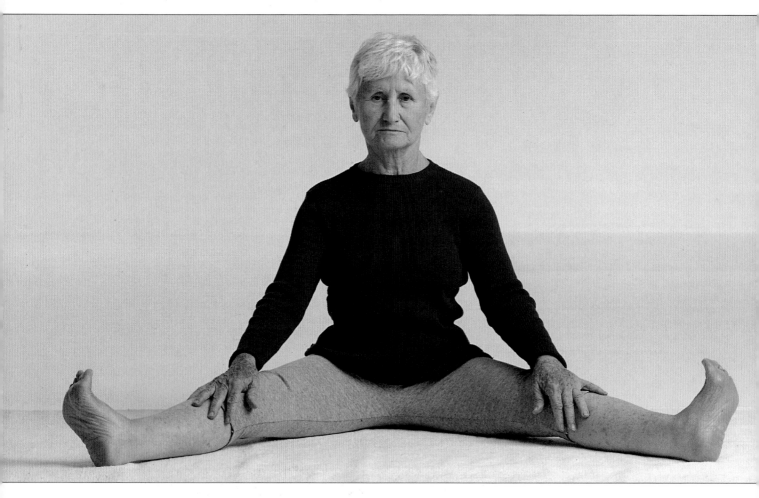

1 *Sit with legs wide apart, your weight evenly distributed on the sitting bones.*

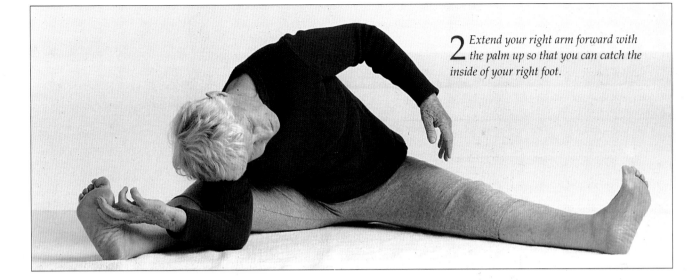

2 Extend your right arm forward with the palm up so that you can catch the inside of your right foot.

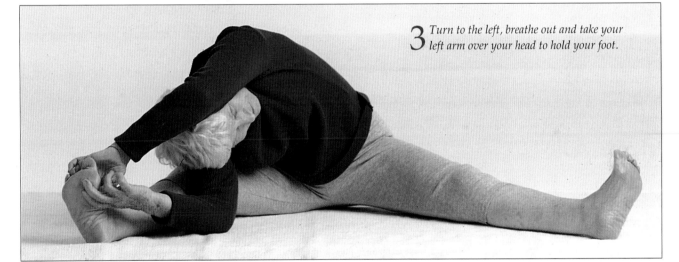

3 Turn to the left, breathe out and take your left arm over your head to hold your foot.

4 On each exhalation you lengthen into the position. Then come up and repeat the position on the other side.

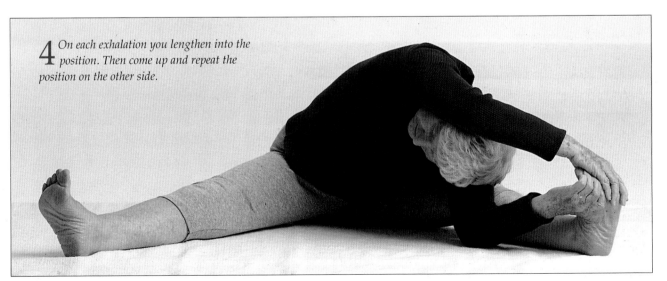

SALUTE to the SUN
SURYA NAMASKAR

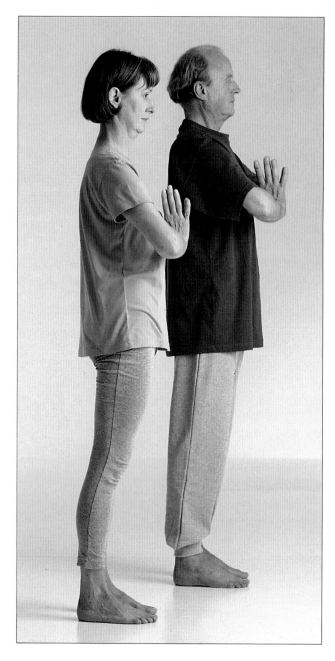

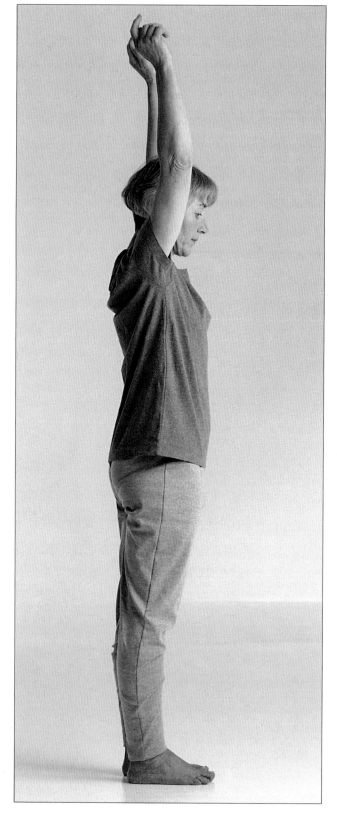

1 *Stand in Mountain (page 18) with your hands folded in the* namaste *position.*

2 *Breathe in and take your arms up. Keep your heels down and relax your shoulders.*

This is a cycle of postures and breathing which has at its center a prostration. It has 12 steps and traditionally it is done 12 times. It is shown here with the right leg moving back and forward. The second time you do it use your left leg so that the cycle is practiced symmetrically. You can also practice more slowly using an exhalation for every movement. Before you try the Salute to the Sun you should be familiar with the individual poses it contains.

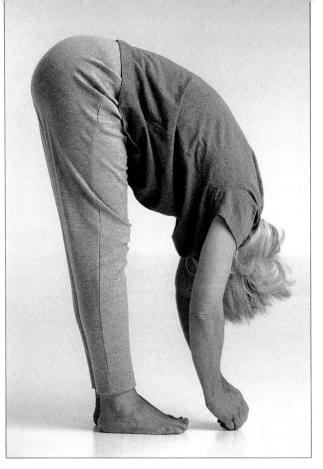

3 *Breathe out and bend forward, keeping your knees straight.*

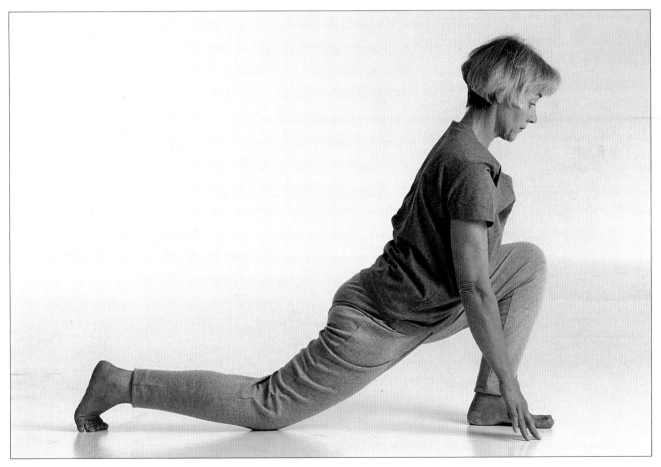

4 *Breathe in, take your right leg back, drop your hips and keep your left heel down.*

SURYA NAMASKAR

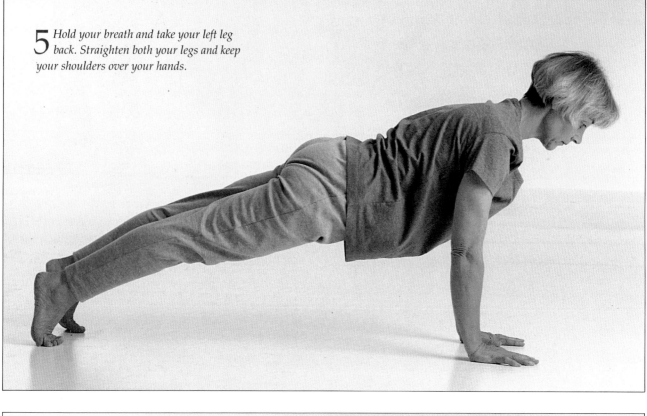

5 *Hold your breath and take your left leg back. Straighten both your legs and keep your shoulders over your hands.*

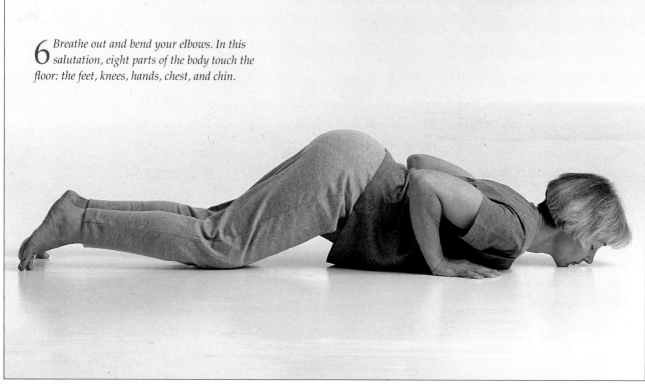

6 *Breathe out and bend your elbows. In this salutation, eight parts of the body touch the floor: the feet, knees, hands, chest, and chin.*

7 *Breathe in and slide forward as you come up into Cobra. Keep your hips down.*

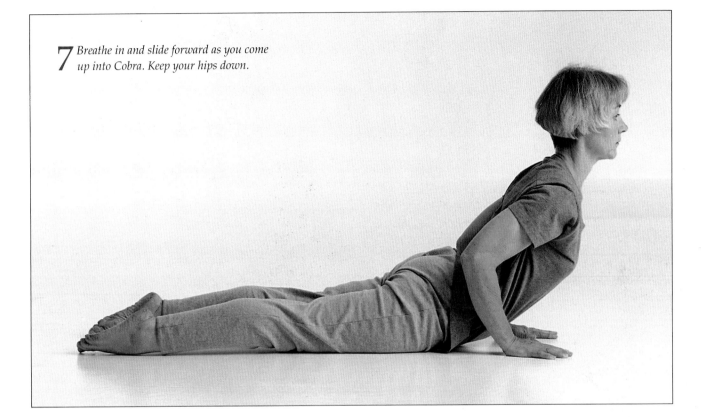

8 *Breathe out and stretch into Dog, taking your heels toward the floor.*

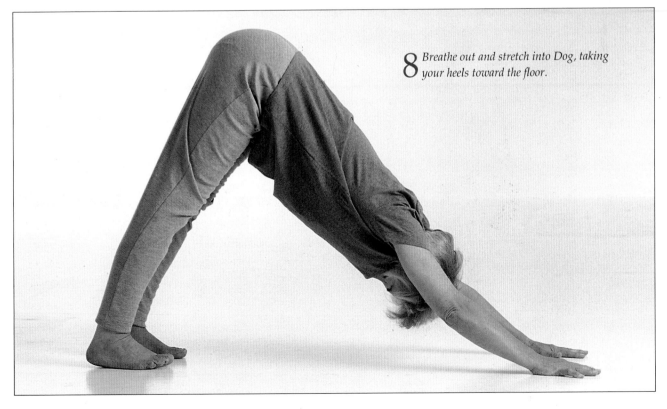

SURYA NAMASKAR

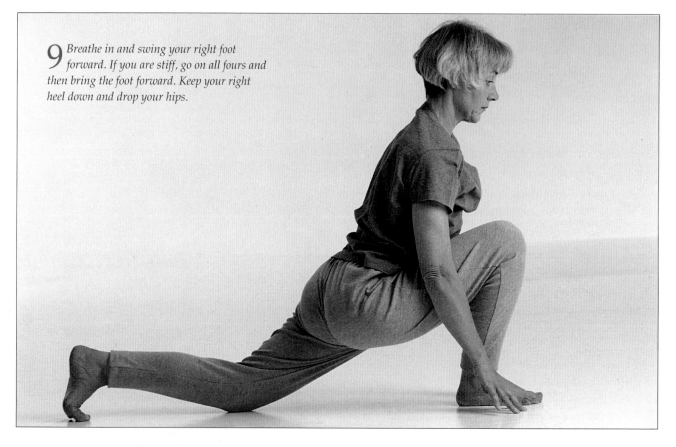

9 *Breathe in and swing your right foot forward. If you are stiff, go on all fours and then bring the foot forward. Keep your right heel down and drop your hips.*

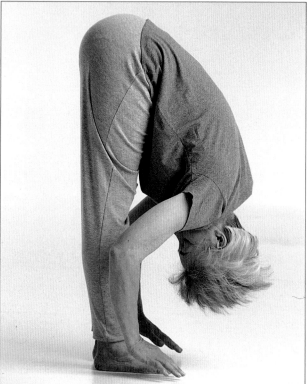

10 *Breathe out, bring the left foot forward, straighten legs so you bend forward.*

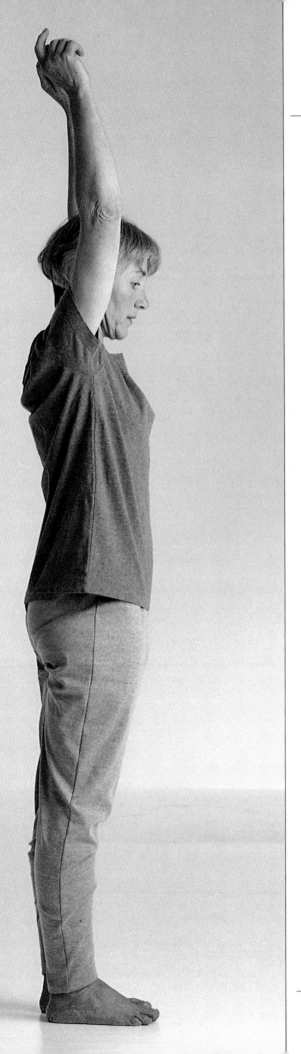

11 *Breathe in; stretch upward with your arms above your head. Keep your weight on your heels and the back of your waist long.*

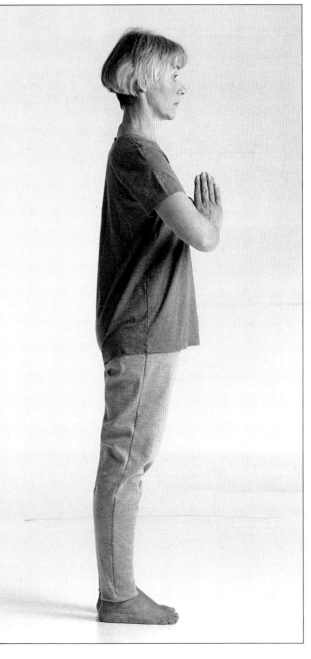

12 *Breathe out and bring your arms down to resume your original position.*

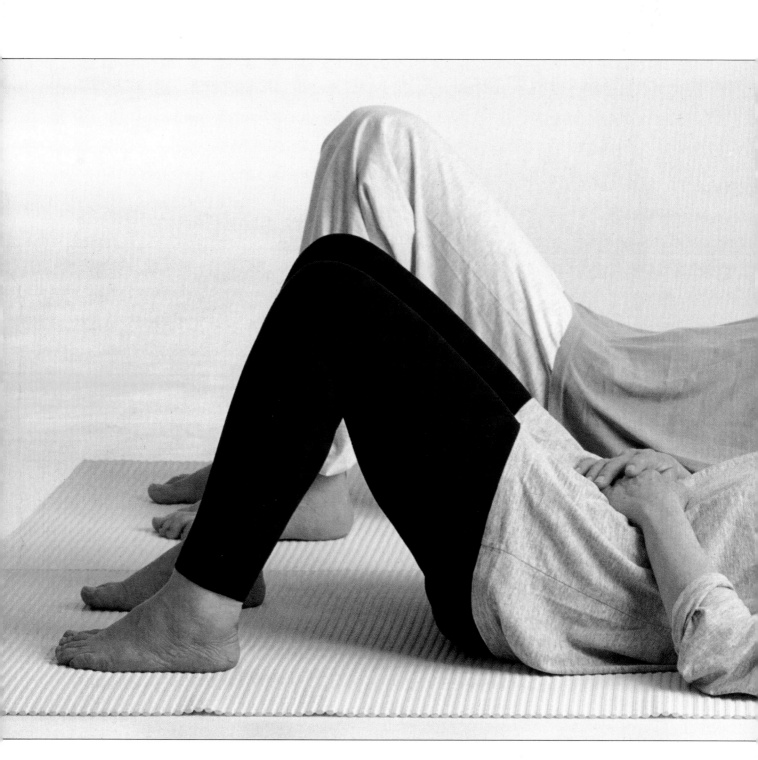

The last three strands of the thread of yoga bring together the body, the mind and the spirit. Tensions in the body dissolve as you relax, and distractions quieten with the rhythm of your breathing. The stillness of your body reflects the silence of your mind. By meditating, all the different facets of yourself are brought to a state of balance and harmony. The spiritual dimension of yoga is as important as the physical; indeed, they are inextricably entwined.

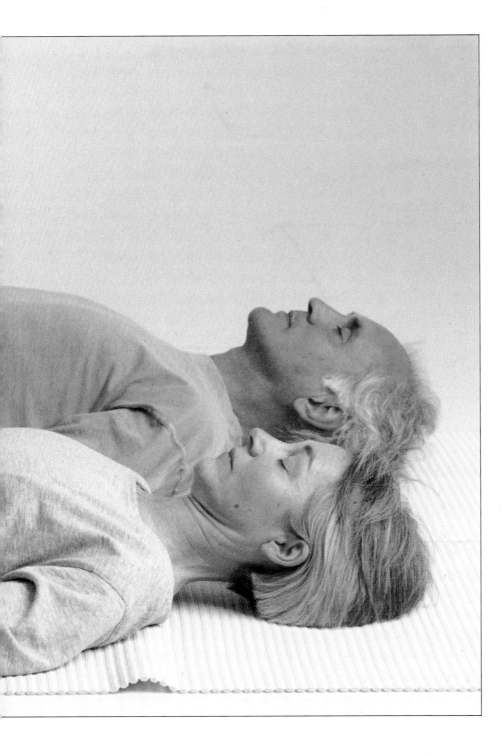

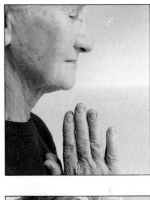

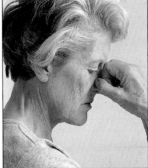

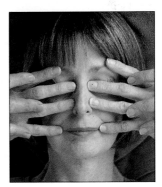

RELAXATION

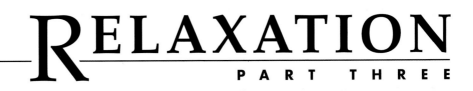

PART THREE

HOW to RELAX

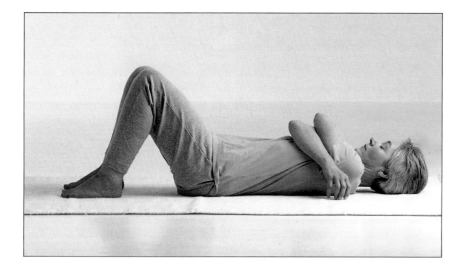

1 *Lie down on your back with your spine as flat as possible and your head straight. Keep your knees bent up with your feet parallel so the back of your waist can touch the floor. Cross your arms over your chest and close your eyes.*

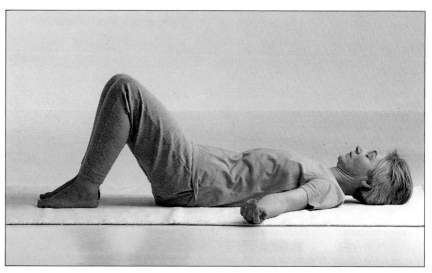

2 *Breathe out and let your arms drop to your sides. Your back should touch the ground from the base of your neck to the bottom of your pelvis. Stay in this position for two to three minutes to allow the back of your waist to lengthen.*

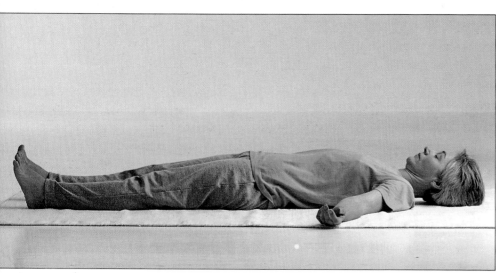

3 *Straighten out your legs into Corpse pose (savasana). As you breathe out let your legs stretch out flat. The back of your waist will come up a little, forming its natural incurve, but your spine will lie longer and flatter than if you had assumed the full position immediately.*

You should allow at least five minutes for relaxation at the end of your practice and once a week stay for 15 to 20 minutes. Relax in a quiet, warm spot. Tensions are usually manifest in the face and hands. Close your eyes and release the tension at the back of the tongue, throat and in the jaw. If you have a tendency to frown, release the tension between your eyebrows. Feel the skin of the palms and finger tips soften. Let the gentle, natural rhythm of your exhaling teach you how to relax. Each time you breathe out let your weight drop down so that your body feels completely supported by the ground beneath you. You may still be a little tense at first but you will become more relaxed with practice.

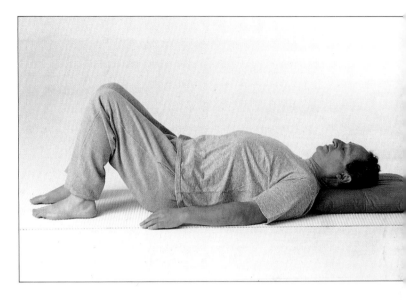

If you are round-shouldered, *put a pillow under your head to relax your neck.*

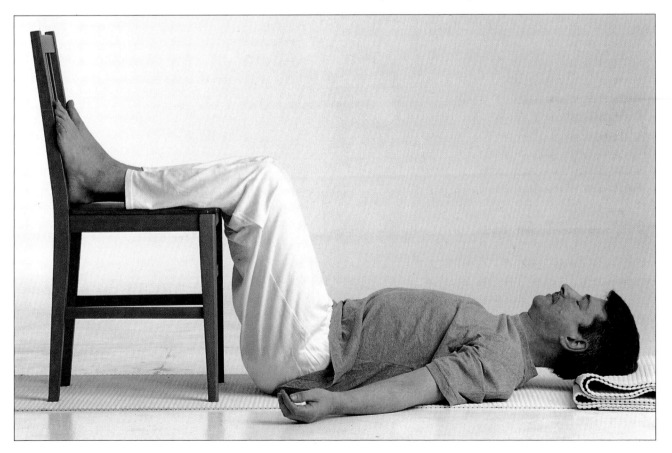

If your lower back aches *owing to tight muscles, raise your legs on to a chair. Your legs should rest comfortably while your back is fully supported by the ground.*

BREATHING
PRANAYAMA

PRANAYAMA MEANS CONTROL (*yama*) of *prana*, which is the life force that energizes every living being – plants, animals and humans. Breath is just one aspect of this. The concept of this life force has a long history. It is breathed into man at creation in the Judaeo-Christian tradition and it is the indwelling divine energy in Hinduism and Buddhism.

Breathing lies on the border between actions over which you have control and those which function automatically. You can slow down your breathing or hold your breath, but only up to a point. You cannot commit suicide by holding your breath as the center in the brain which controls your breathing automatically takes over and you breathe to survive. However you can hurt yourself by breathing too forcefully or holding your breath for too long. Breathing has to be practiced slowly and carefully with an understanding of how your body works.

The main muscle of breathing is the diaphragm, which lies across the bottom of the ribcage dividing the chest from the abdomen. It is slightly domed upwards like an open umbrella and is higher at the front, where it attaches to the bottom of the breastbone, than at the back, where it attaches to the lower ribs. The diaphragm contracts in the center and descends when you breathe in, so that the volume in the chest is increased and your lungs fill with air. When you breathe out the diaphragm relaxes and goes up and the volume of the chest is decreased. This means that as you breathe the pressures in the chest and abdomen change, affecting the functioning of the heart and circulation and many other systems in the body.

To work properly the diaphragm needs to be anchored by its long muscle fibers at the back.

These fibers descend far below the back ribs, reaching down the front of the spine almost to the top of the pelvis. Posture is therefore all-important when doing any breathing exercises. To accommodate the expansion of the lungs the ribcage needs to be elastic and the abdominal muscles and pelvic floor have to be strong to resist the increase of pressure in the abdomen.

Breathing is a continual rhythmic action which needs all the muscles to be toned and elastic so that it becomes part of the balance as you move, stand and sit. To practice the *asanas*

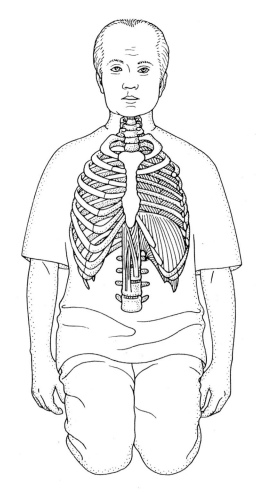

This diagram of the chest illustrates the position of the diaphragm in relation to the ribs and spine.

correctly all movement should be in tune with the action of breathing.

When you sit properly the muscles which support the cavities of the chest and abdomen can relax and contract efficiently as you breathe, their action helping to maintain the alignment of your spine. The action of these muscles in the pelvic floor, abdomen and neck is described as a lock (*bandha*). The *moola bandha* is the tightening of the pelvic floor and lower abdomen, the *uddiyana bandha* is when the abdomen from breastbone to pubic bone is pulled back towards the spine on exhalation and the *jalandhara bandha* is the extension of the back of the head upward as the chin is drawn in. When you sit well, these locks happen automatically without any feeling of strain.

Just as some people begin yoga practice with bad posture that has to be understood and worked with, others have to learn to relax and change patterns of breathing. Tensions and stresses, which affect posture, also influence the way we breathe and have a profound effect on the way you feel physically and psychologically. Rapid, shallow breathing is both the result of anxiety and the cause of a restless state.

When you practice *pranayama* each breath can bring you closer to a state of equilibrium. Like the *asanas, pranayama* is a voyage of self-discovery. However, its exercises tune the body at a finer level as they work not only on the rhythms of the breath, the circulatory and nervous systems but also on your ability to concentrate. *Pranayama* is a far more delicate exercise than the *asanas*: remember that the eventual aim is silence and concentration. Any movements that make you feel anxious, strained or even aggressive should not be attempted.

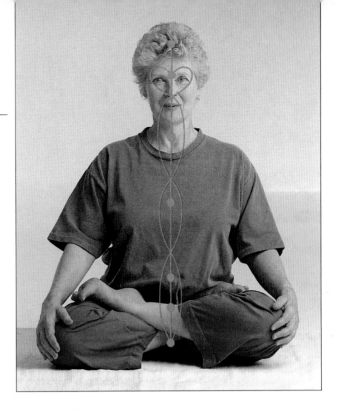

The chakras lie along the line of the spine. When you sit, this vertical central axis should be aligned with the pull of gravity.

Hatha yoga and the concept of the chakras

In the Hatha yoga tradition the body consists of five different layers, of varying degrees of density. The physical body we experience with our senses is just one of these. In the subtle body, of which you are normally unaware, *prana* is channeled along paths known as *nadis*. One of the functions of *asanas* is to clear these so energy can flow freely, balancing the *ha* (sun) and *tha* (moon) energy. There are a great many of these channels; the two principals being the *pingala*, carrying the sun energy and the *ida*, carrying the moon. These spiral up the body crossing the *susumna*, a channel which approximates the line of the spine. This channel is blocked at the base in most people and the psychic energy therein (known as *kundalini*, the sleeping serpent goddess) lies dormant. In Hatha yoga the ultimate aim of *asanas* and *pranayama* is to awaken this potential force. As it moves up, energy centers (*chakras* – wheels) lying along the *susumna* are activated to bring a new state of consciousness, physically and mentally.

FINDING the BREATH

AND HOW TO SIT

LIE DOWN ON YOUR BACK with your knees bent up. If this is not comfortable, put your legs on a chair and your head on a cushion (page 111).

Put your hands on your lower abdomen with the thumbs on your navel and the little fingers toward the pubic bone. Stay quiet for a minute or two and breathe gently. Breathe out slowly; your abdomen should go down beneath your hands towards your spine as you do this. Wait and let the breath come in slowly; feel your abdomen rise up again as you breathe in.

Practice breathing like this and feel the rise and fall of the abdomen while keeping your shoulders, upper body and neck as relaxed as possible. Don't try to "take" the breath, forcefully pushing out your chest and arching

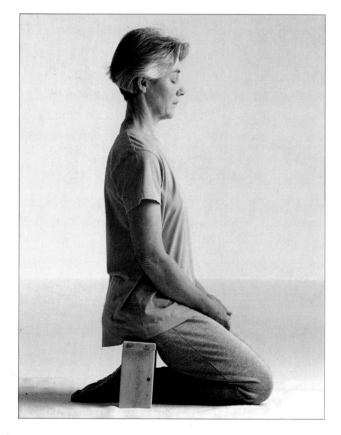

A comfortable way to sit for breathing is to use a meditation stool.

your waist. This action of the abdomen will happen automatically for some, but for others (particularly those with bad posture) it will be more difficult. In this case, practice briefly several times a day until you get the rhythm of breathe out, stomach in, breathe in, stomach out.

Sitting for *pranayama* or meditation
When you sit, the base of the pose, the pelvis, has to be straight, with the two sitting bones going down towards the ground. Then your spine can balance easily in its four curves and the muscles of the *bandhas* function properly. If your pelvis tilts forward, your waist curves in too far and there will be a downward pressure in the lower abdomen and pelvic floor. If your pelvis tips backward the curve of your waist collapses back and your spine is dragged down, rounding your back and constricting your chest.

By far the easiest way to sit properly is on the floor, either in Lotus (page 74), Half-Lotus (page 28) or Diamond (page 62). In these positions the pelvis can stay straight as the spine lengthens and balances as you breathe. You need to be supple to fold your legs into these positions, but if you can, it is more comfortable to sit like this for a long time than it is to sit in a chair. Ordinary cross-legged poses and straight-legged poses such as Sitting Stretch (page 78), Cobbler's Pose (page 68) and Hero (page 64) tilt the pelvis and are unsuitable for any length of time.

If you have difficulty staying in Diamond you can put a blanket under your feet and/or a cushion over your heels. You can also use a meditation stool, which is a little wooden bridge that fits across your ankles as you kneel (*see left*).

If you need to sit in a chair, be sure that it is the right height so that you can sit straight with your thighs horizontal and your feet on the floor. If the chair is too low, sit on a cushion; if it is too high, put a stool or a book under your feet. Ideally, your spine should not rest against the back of the chair, but should lengthen upward and adjust as you breathe. However, if you need support, make sure your chair is vertical and that the base of your spine touches it.

To find the action of the breath when sitting
Sit down in whichever position is comfortable. Make sure that you are straight with your weight distributed evenly on both sitting bones. Relax your shoulders and your arms and put your hands on your lower abdomen as you did when you were lying down. The abdominal muscles should tighten and go in when you breathe out and relax as you breathe in. Keep the inhalation passive and gentle.

If you are sitting correctly, at the end of the exhalation the three *bandhas* can function, the pelvic floor and abdomen will be contracted and your spine, from the tail to the top of the neck, will be straight and tall with your chin slightly drawn inward. As you focus on the rhythm of your breathing, you will become aware of the moment in the exhalation when tension is released and you automatically "let go", as in the moment during a yawn when you want to stretch. This release with the flow of the breath is the impulse that takes you into the *asanas* and is the key to relaxation and quiet.

Mudras (seals) are positions which close circuits of energy or activity. These are calming, steadying techniques that you can use to help you quieten down as you sit for breathing.
Khekari mudra Turn your tongue back so that the tip points toward the back of your throat and the underside touches the roof of the mouth. This helps to relax your jaw and position your head in the right place at the top of your spine.
Jnana mudra Touch the tip of your index finger to the tip of your thumb while resting your hands on your knees. This relaxes tension in the palms of your hands and symbolizes the union of the individual with the infinite.

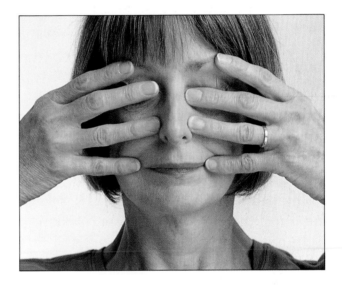

To relax for the breathing exercises, do sanmukhi mudra.

Sanmukhi mudra Close your eyes and very gently place your hands over your face with your thumbs closing your ears. The soft pads of your fingers rest on your eyebrows, eyelids and the corners of your nose and mouth. As you breathe out, allow your face to widen. This will relax your mouth, eyes, and the frown lines between your eyebrows.

When you lie down to relax you can get a similar effect by putting a small bag filled with rice over your eyes. The rice will fall to each end of the bag, helping your face to relax. Don't fill the bag too full. There should be no direct pressure on the eyes and if you have had any eye problems, consult your doctor first.

BREATHING EXERCISES

IT IS IMPORTANT TO PRACTICE breathing exercises regularly so try to set aside at least ten minutes at the same time each day. Don't practice on a full stomach, or on a completely empty one. Sit up with your pelvis straight and your spine and head erect, then breathe through your nose unless otherwise instructed. Practice new techniques for a few breaths only and don't do any exercise for more than five minutes, except for the simple *ujjayi* breathing. Never force the breathing as some exercises may simply not be appropriate for you.

Cleansing breath (*kapalabhati*)   This is usually done before the other breathing exercises as it expels stale air from the lungs, stabilizes the sitting position and relaxes the upper body.

Breathe out and in gently. Then breathe out by pulling in the abdominal muscle quickly. Release the abdomen immediately to let you breathe in and repeat up to five times. Fill the lungs by slowly releasing the abdominal muscle. Repeat up to three times. Start with five to ten quick exhalations and then one long inhalation. Increase the number of exhalations until you can do 60 at a time (this will take some months). Practice gently. If you have problems with your heart, blood pressure or eyes take medical advice before doing this breathing exercise.

Simple deep breathing (*ujjayi*)   This slow, rhythmic breathing is the key to sitting still and in silence, but its simplicity makes it difficult. You have to concentrate and allow the breath to continually adjust and balance the sitting position in accordance with the pull of gravity.

Breathe out, slowly letting the abdomen draw inwards toward the spine. Let your breath come in gently and without effort. Don't try to lift the chest as this will merely shorten the back and block the lungs. This gentle, deep breathing teaches the perfect sitting posture, which in turn shows you how to breathe.

Interval breathing (*viloma*)   This is a way of adjusting the length of the breath. Pausing during the inhalation is helpful if you are feeling low or depressed. Practice on alternate breaths to begin with. When the technique becomes familiar you can do it on every breath.

1. *Interval breathing on the exhalation*   Breathe in slowly. Relax your shoulders and pause briefly. Breathe out a little and pause. Continue, pausing for one second and with equal intervals of exhalation. Do not pause at the end of the exhalation but relax and breathe in normally.

2. *Interval breathing on the inhalation*   Breathe out then breathe in a little. Pause, breathe in, then pause again. Continue, pausing for one second and with equal intervals of inhalation. Pause at the end of the breath and breathe out normally.

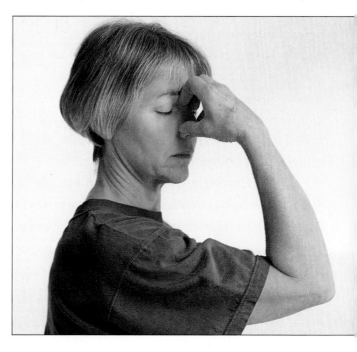

To clear the nasal passages, pinch your nostrils and breathe alternately through each one.

Holding the breath (*kumbhaka*)   Holding the breath is an experience of silence and stillness; it has nothing to do with "holding tight" or trying to see how long you can go without breathing.

Hold the breath at the end of the "in" breath then breathe out slowly so that the exhalation is twice the length of the inhalation. Practice this ratio of one to two before attempting to hold your breath. Breathe in, relax your shoulders and face as you hold your breath, then breathe out slowly. Take one or two normal breaths before repeating the cycle. The maximum time you should hold your breath is three times the length of the inhalation.

Alternate nostril breathing (*nadi sodhana*)   This clears the channels by alternating the breath through the right and left nostrils. If it makes your shoulders tense and disturbs the way you sit, then this is not for you at the moment.

To close the nostrils use a little pressure on the side of the nose where the cartilage meets the bone. The thumb of the right hand closes the right nostril and the little and fourth fingers close the left nostril (*see left*).

Sit straight and bring your right hand to your face without tensing the shoulder. Close the left nostril; breathe out through the right. Breathe in through the right nostril, close both nostrils, release the left side and breathe out and then in through the left. Repeat and continue changing channels at the end of the "in" breath and finish by breathing out of the right side, then breath in with both nostrils.

Lion breath (*simhasana*)   Here, air is breathed in through the nose and breathed out along the tongue, sounding like a roar. Sit up straight, breathe in, pull your chin in and put your tongue out so that the tip touches your chin; at

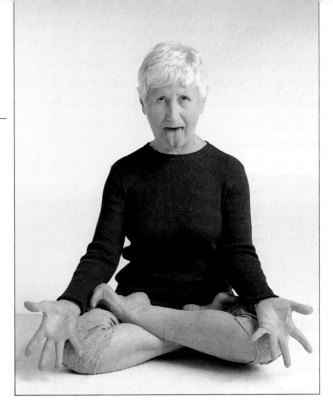

The lion breath is an invigorating exercise that will wake you up.

the same time look up to your eyebrows. Breathe out quickly though your open mouth. Do for a maximum of three times; do not do it if you have high blood pressure or eye problems.

Buzzing breath (*bhamari*)   This is a relaxing and energizing exercise which also makes you alert and awake. Sit straight and breathe in normally. As you breathe out make a buzzing sound by bringing your lips together to vibrate. Take the vibration back so that you can feel it at the back of your head and neck. With practice you will be able to feel it in your chest and at the back of your ribs. At first, just try this on alternate out-breaths. The more you relax, the further down your spine you will feel the interior buzzing.

Aum   When you turn the vibration breath into an "mmmm" sound you may, if you wish, sound the syllable "aum" as you breathe out, ending the vowel sound with the vibration "mmmm". Aum is used as a *mantra*, and is the vibration of all created things. Hence its sounding is a serious practice and something not to be done trivially, but with reverence. "All speech is held together by aum" – *Chandogga Upanishad*.

MEDITATION

AT THE END OF PRANAYAMA you are sitting straight, still and with your attention focused on your breathing and undistracted by sight or sound. This is the beginning of meditation. In yoga, meditation is the stilling of the mind. It is not thinking about an object or pondering on a problem or using your imagination.

To be still and silent sounds very simple, but it is difficult for us because human beings are complex creatures and both the body and the mind tend to be restless. Through the *asanas* you

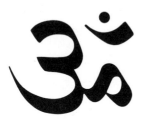

The 'aum' is a popular mantra for meditating.

learn how to sit straight, stable and relaxed without being tense and rigid or collapsing and dozing off. *Pranayama* also teaches you to find the balance between restlessness and inertia, helping you let go of anxieties and worries as you focus on the breath without letting yourself follow distracting thoughts. So meditation which involves the mind is a natural progression from the earlier physical steps of yoga practice. Yoga poses, relaxation and breathing can be practiced by anyone, at any time of their life with no other goal than the health, energy and freedom from stress that they bring. Meditation cannot be practiced for these reasons alone. It is part of a religious path and the idea of material gain, even health and equilibrium, is incompatible with its practice.

Concentration (*Dharana*)

As with *asanas* and *pranayama*, meditation takes time and practice. To begin with, try sitting still and silent for a few minutes at the end of your *pranayama* exercises before you lie down to relax.

Focus on the natural rhythm of your breathing. Allow yourself a set time to do this, so that you don't just give up when you first become distracted. Distracting thoughts are bound to come when you try to be still and silent but you don't have to hold on to them and let them take you over. If you concentrate on the gentle rhythm of the inflow and outflow of your breath this will become like a continuous thread that you can follow through the maze of your thoughts to an increasing center of quiet within you. If you find that you have lost the thread and wandered off, gently detach yourself from the distraction and refocus on your breathing.

To begin with, this can be extremely difficult and even five minutes can seem like an eternity when you are restless; with practice it becomes much easier. Later on you can increase the time you sit, but you should keep to a regular discipline. It is the regular, daily practice that is important. Sitting for a long time one day when you feel calm and collected and giving up when your attention keeps wandering on the following day will only tend to make you more scattered. It is important to keep to a balanced routine so set a maximum as well as a minimum time for meditating. Meditation twice a day for between 20 and 30 minutes is the ideal. Early in the morning, when the day's distractions have not had time to take over, and after practicing *pranayama*, when you are naturally quiet and focused, are the best times.

Besides concentrating on your breathing there are other methods you can use to quieten your thoughts when you meditate. You can concentrate by repeating a word or sound, through visualization or through focusing on parts of your body such as the heart.

Unfortunately there are groups and cults marketing such methods as the panacea for all ills or as the pathways to exotic experiences such as levitation. Just as *asanas* and *pranayama* practiced foolishly can pull muscles or disturb your state of well-being, practicing unsuitable meditation techniques can have adverse effects mentally. So if you want to learn to use a technique other than the simple concentration on the breath, then exercise your judgement and common sense and find a method that feels right for you, in keeping with your cultural and religious roots. As in *asanas* and *pranayama* you should start from where you are and not try to impose some strange and alien discipline on yourself. Meditation is a continuous lifelong practice. Once you have established a way of practicing you should stay with it and practice regularly. The method you use will form an important part of your life, so you need to take your time and think carefully before choosing the right way for you.

In most major religions, there are words or phrases which are used as a way of calming the mind and which hold your attention at a deeper and deeper level as you practice concentrating on them. These words or sounds are known in yoga as *mantras*, and this method of meditation is one of the most widely used at present. Traditionally, this way of meditation is started and continued under the supervision of a teacher. If you meet with problems, you need someone to turn to for advice and, although by its nature meditation is usually practiced alone, the support of a group is helpful.

Any form of yoga, whether it is *asana*, *pranayama* or meditation, brings increased health, sensitivity and energy but this should not make you feel "different" or isolate you from others. Rather, it is a question of increasing your potential in every possible way, regardless of age, and of giving you the ability to live life to its fullest. Being in touch with other people who are doing the same thing can be inspiring.

Any method of concentration will eventually involve all your attention until you are completely and continually absorbed. This is meditation (*dhyana*), by which you pass beyond the sound, image or breath, through the looking glass of the mind with its reflections, to the spirit that lies within and contemplation (*samadhi*).

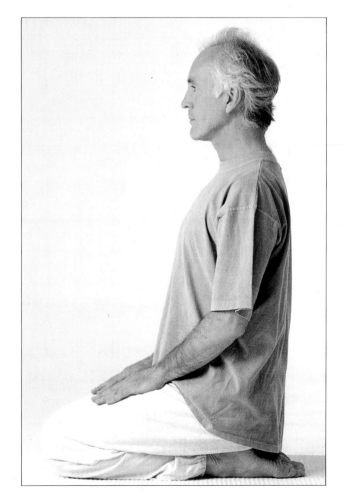

Sit in a suitable pose, such as Diamond (page 62), before meditating.

PROGRAMMES

INTRODUCTION

As you get older regular practice is even more important. It will be ultimately more satisfying, and it will also help prevent the aching or injury that might be caused by sudden exercise. Put aside a set time each day when you intend to practise. Don't exercise on a full stomach or late at night. Thirty minutes a day will be ample to start with, but even ten minutes is beneficial, if that is all you can manage. Find a quiet place with a level non-slip surface (you may need to use a mat). Wear loose stretchy clothes and keep a sweater handy for relaxation. Do it in bare feet so that you can stretch your toes. You will need a blanket for the sitting and inverted poses and a chair. You may also need a belt and two cushions if you are stiff. If you have any specific medical problems, consult your doctor before starting the postures and breathing exercises.

To begin with, keep to the set programs given below. Warm up with simple poses before trying the more challenging part of your practice and leave time at the end to relax. The postures have to balance each other so the spine stretches evenly. Thus forward bends are balanced with backbends, for example, and active poses with quieter, calming ones. Always stretch both sides in asymmetric poses, and practice breathing and relaxation from day one.

Programs The first programme is designed for people who are very stiff. Beginners who are moderately stiff should first do the standard beginners' program then interchange with the alternative beginners' program. Gradually you can progress to the standard maintenance routines. The general programs are planned to last about 30 minutes and do not include Headstand, Lotus or the more intense forward or backbends. If you want to do these then you need to go slowly, building up your practice to at least an hour a day, not including the time needed for breathing and relaxation.

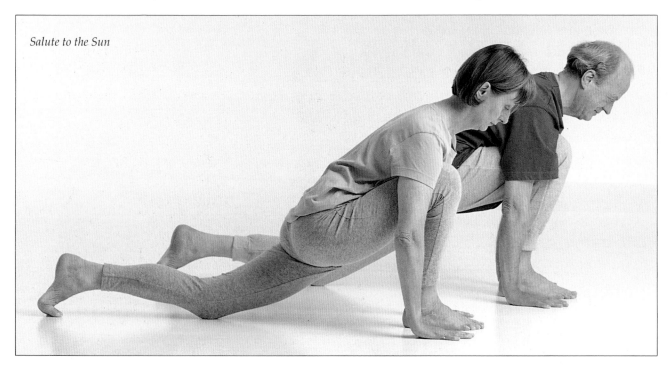

Salute to the Sun

BEGINNERS' ROUTINES

PROGRAM FOR THE VERY STIFF

Practice little and often if mobility is a problem, preferably two or three times a day. This program starts and ends with sitting up tall and breathing deeply. The time it takes will depend on your mobility and stamina. If the standing poses Mountain and Triangle are too difficult, then omit these and do more of the lying floor stretches (pages 58–59) instead.

Sit straight in a chair and find your breath	114
Stretch up, one arm at a time	40
Stretch forward to second chair	42
Sitting stretch to floor	42
Sitting twist	41
Sitting shoulder stretch with belt	41
Sitting forward stretch with legs apart	42
Mountain	18
Triangle, *step 1 only*	28
Bridge with head on pillow	90
Stretch arms over head, arms on pillows	58
Leg stretches, *step 1 only*	54
Relax, legs on chair and head on pillow	110
Sitting straight in a chair, practise slow, simple *ujjayi* breathing for ten breaths	116

STANDARD BEGINNERS' PROGRAM

The beginners' routine starts with simple standing poses to make you grounded and balanced. Stop if you feel any strain or discomfort.

Mountain *and* Tree	18
Foot exercises	125
Cow *and* Eagle, arms only	70
Standing Forward Bend to chair	20
Standing Twist	30
Warrior, *step 1*	32
Child	66
Dog	67
Half-Shoulder Stand against a wall	45
Plough with chair	48
Leg stretches, *step 1*	54
Floor Twist	56
Diamond	62
Ujjayi deep breathing	116
Relax	110

ALTERNATIVE BEGINNERS' PROGRAM

Alternate with standard beginners' program after four weeks of daily practice. When you have warmed up try the Half-Shoulder Stand then the floor poses before you quieten down for relaxation and breathing.

Mountain	18
Triangle Forward Bend	24
Triangle	26
Wide Angle Pose to chair	22
Diamond	62
Child	66
Dog	67
Half-Shoulder Stand against a wall	46
Plough with chair	48
Floor Twist	56
Floor poses	58
Five *kapalabhati* then *ujjayi* deep breathing	116
Sit still for five minutes	

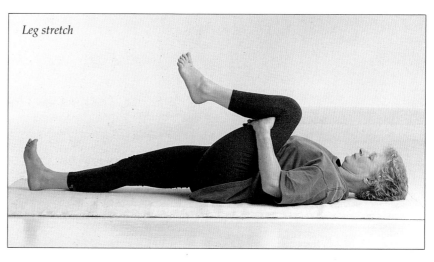

Leg stretch

MAINTENANCE ROUTINES

After four months of practice you can gradually introduce new *asanas* to cover the next four programs. Follow the plan of standing poses, then shoulder stands, floor poses and sitting poses for programs A and B. When you have been practicing these programs for several months you can start to learn the Salute to the Sun and do program C once or twice a week.

STANDARD ROUTINE A

Mountain *and* Tree	18
Standing Forward Bend	20
Triangle	26
Standing Twist	30
Wide Angle Pose	22
Child	66
Dog	67
Angle Pose Twist	38
Locust	88
Sitting stretch	78
Shoulder Stand	44
Plough	48
Leg stretches	54
Floor Twist	56
Diamond for breathing	62
Kapalabhati gently ten strokes three times. Then *ujjayi* breathing	114
Sit still for five minutes	
Relax	110

STANDARD ROUTINE B

Mountain	18
Triangle Forward Bend	24
Warrior	32
Standing Twist	30
Standing Forward Bend	20
Shoulder Stand	44
Plough	48
Shoulder Stand, one leg down	46
Bridge	90
Half-Bound Angle	80
Half-Hero	81
Sage	94
Sage Twist	96
Sitting Stretch	78
Cobbler's Pose, *step 1*	68
Lotus, *step 1*	74
Introduce interval breathing on the exhalation	116
Sit still for ten minutes	
Relax	110

STANDARD ROUTINE C

Salute to the Sun	102
Angle Pose Twist	38
Shoulder Stand	44
Plough	48
Floor Twist	56
Diamond or Half-Lotus for breathing	62, 74
Kapalabhati gently for 10 strokes then *ujjayi* breathing	116
Sit still for ten minutes	

STANDARD ROUTINE D

This program starts with floor poses and is good if you have had to leave your practice until late. Don't do this program more than twice in one week as you need the standing poses for stamina and energy.

Lie flat, knees bent up, breathing	110
Leg stretches	54
Child	66
Dog	67
Hero	64
Forward Angle Pose	82
Cobbler's Pose	68
Wide Angle Twist	100
Sitting Stretch	78
Shoulder Stand	44
Plough	48
Bridge	90
Floor Twist	56
Lie flat, knees bent up, breathing	110
Relax	110
Practice *pranayama* sitting up in Half-Lotus with your back to the wall after you have rested.	74

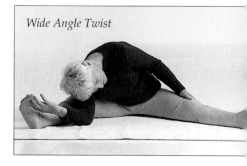

Wide Angle Twist

ADVANCED ROUTINES

These programs take over 30 minutes and are suitable for people who have practiced regularly for a year or more. The increased stretch required should be a natural extension of the simple poses. Omit poses marked * if you find them difficult. Introduce variations for Headstand, Shoulder Stand and Lotus when the basic pose is stable and comes easily.

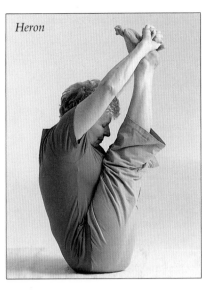
Heron

ADVANCED ROUTINE A

Mountain	18
Standing Forward Bend	20
Triangle & twist	26
Angle Pose Twist	38
Half-Moon & twist	34
Child	66
Headstand*	50
More Headstands*	52
Dog	67
Shoulder Stand	44
Plough	48
Bridge	90
Wheel*	91
Sitting Stretch	78
Half-Bound Angle	80
Half-Hero	81
Sage	94
Heron	85
Diamond for breathing	62
Relax	110

ADVANCED ROUTINE B

Salute to the Sun six times	102
Angle Pose Twist	38
Crane	36
Child	66
Headstand	50
Dog	67
Shoulder Stand	44
Plough	48
More Shoulder Stands*	46
Bridge	90
Wheel*	91
Forward Angle Pose	82
Wide Angle Twist	100
Hero	64
Lotus*	74
More Lotus poses*	76
Cobbler's Pose	68
Breathing in Diamond or Lotus	62, 74
Relax	110

ADVANCED ROUTINE C

morning

Mountain *and* Tree	18
Half-Lotus Standing	28
Warrior	32
Standing Twist	30
Wide Angle Pose	22
Dog	67
Locust	66
Bow	88
Wheel*	90
Sage	94
Tortoise*	86
Sleeping Pose*	60
Sage Twist	96
Half-Sage Twist	98
Diamond or Lotus for breathing	62, 74
Relax	110

evening

Headstand*	50
More Headstands*	52
Dog	67
Shoulder Stand	44
More Shoulder Stands	46
Plough	48
Sitting Stretch	78
Hero	64
Cow	70
Cobbler's Pose	68
Lotus for breathing	74
Relax	110

PROBLEM ROUTINES

These are short programs to deal with specific problems. Practice the appropriate program to loosen up before you do your regular routine.

QUIET, RELAXING ROUTINE

This is a marvellous routine to do when you are tired and stiff, after a journey, a heavy day, or before you go to sleep at night. It can also be used as a preliminary exercise for other programs; in which case omit the breathing and relaxation section as you will do this at the end of the main program.

Lie on back, knees bent, for five minutes	110
Stretch your arms over your head	58
Leg stretches	54
Floor Twist	56
Child with head supported	66
Dog	67
Diamond for breathing	62
Kapalabhati gently 20 times then 20 deep breaths. If stressed, *viloma* on the exhalation	116
Relax	110

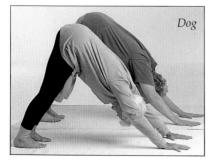

Dog

ROUTINE FOR STIFF HIPS A

This is a gentle routine for stiff hips. Stay in each pose and let go in the hips as you breathe out. Gradually increase the time you hold the position.

Lie on your back with your legs apart up a wall	54
Bend knees	54
Sit with your back to a wall, legs wide apart	82
Half-Bound Angle, cushion under bent knee	78
Cobbler's Pose by wall, knees supported	64
Hero with cushion	60
Sitting Stretch	78

ROUTINE FOR STIFF HIPS B

This is a more active program to help you stay mobile. If one hip is stiffer than the other, practice for longer on the side you find difficult. The movement must be in the hips and not strain the knees. Release the stiffness as you breathe out and do not force the pose.

Hero, on a cushion if your sitting bones don't touch the floor	64
Monkey, *step 1*	72
Cow, legs only	70
Leg stretches	54
Cobbler's Pose: your back should be supported by a wall with cushions under your thighs	68

QUICK RELEASES FOR TENSE SHOULDERS

If you find your shoulders and upper back are feeling stiff and tense but you do not have time to do a full routine, try one of the following asanas to release the tension:

Standing Forward Bend to chair	20
Dog	67
Standing Twist	30
Angle Pose Twist, *step 1*	38
Sage	92
Cow, arms only while standing.	70
Eagle	71
Wide Angle Pose, stretch forward to a chair	22
Floor pose, arms over head	58
Chair pose twist	41
Chair shoulder stretch with belt	41

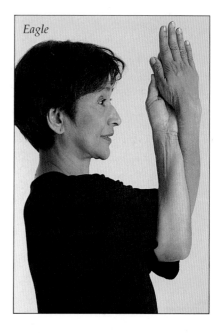

Eagle

ROUTINE FOR SHOULDERS

Do this program to release tension in your shoulders. If you have difficulty sleeping follow this program, then practice the quiet, relaxing routine (page 124).

BACKACHE

All poses should stretch your spine. Do the beginners' programs on page 121 and use a chair for any forward bends. Repeat twice a day.

QUICK SALUTE TO THE SUN

This is an invigorating way of stretching the spine when you have little time, or are not yet able to do the full Salute to the Sun. Practice steps 1–4 (pages 102–103), breathe out, take your left leg back and go into step 8 (page 109) and complete the cycle. Repeat on the other side.

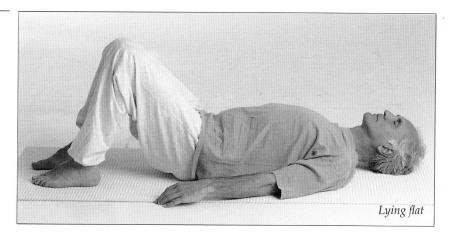

Lying flat

FEET

Everybody needs to stretch their feet to keep healthy. The way your feet work affects your posture, comfort and appearance. This is a program of foot exercises you can do before your yoga practice, or at the end of a hard day. Take your shoes off and stretch your feet to restore your energy before you relax. It is essential to work in bare feet.

KNEES

If you have knee problems practice stretches for the hips and feet as well as this program, as these may strain your knee joints.

HANDS

In all the poses where the hands are on the floor, extend your fingers so the centre of your palm stretches. When you do the namaste *position stretch your hands so that your fingers touch each other from base to tip, as well as the palms.*

INDEX

ACKNOWLEDGEMENTS

Editorial Director Sandy Carr   **Art Director** Jason Vrakas
Designer Victor-Manuel Ibañez   **Assistant Editor** Sara Harper
Design Assistant Adelle Morris
Assistant to Sandra Lousada Gemma Day   **Make-up** Ellen Kramer
Illustrations Annabel Milne   **Indexer** Naomi Good
Production Charles James   **Desktop Publishing** Jonathan Harley

Picture acknowledgements
Gautama the Buddha, Nepalese gilt-copper figure The Bridgeman
Art Library
Section from painting *Diwali, or Feast of Light: ladies performing ritual.*
Lucknow, 1760. The Victoria and Albert Museum

The author and publishers would like to thank all those who helped in
the preparation of this book, in particular, the models who took part in
the photography sessions. The models were Tony Anholt,
Marah Dickson-Wright, Catherine James, Cathy Janson, Leila Keyes,
Rosie Lovat, Patrick Moorsom, Benjamin Pogrund, Margot St Jacques,
Vanda Scaravelli, Terence Stamp and James Stuart.
They would also like to thank Joan Price's Face Place for doing the
manicures and pedicures.

ABOUT THE AUTHOR

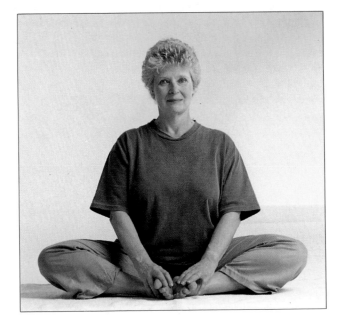

Mary Stewart has been teaching yoga for more than 20 years to private clients, classes and teachers of yoga all over the world. She has developed methods based on breathing following the work of Vanda Scaravelli and believes that you can benefit from yoga well into old age. She began to learn yoga from a book and feels this is a good way of being introduced to yoga. This is her fifth book: her previous publications include Yoga for Children.